Clinical Skills Manual for Pediatric Nursing
Caring For Children

Fourth Edition

Ruth C. McGillis Bindler, PhD, RNC

Professor, Washington State University
Intercollegiate College of Nursing
Spokane, Washington

Jane W. Ball, DrPH, RN, CPNP

Emergency Medical Services and Trauma Systems Consultant
Gaithersburg, Maryland

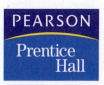

PEARSON

Prentice
Hall

Upper Saddle River, New Jersey 07458

Library of Congress Cataloging-in-Publication Data

Bindler, Ruth C. McGillis.
    Clinical skills manual for pediatric nursing / Ruth C. Bindler, Jane W. Ball. — 4th ed.
        p. cm.
    Includes bibliographical references.
    ISBN 0-13-613554-4
    1. Pediatric nursing—Handbooks, manuals, etc. I. Ball, Jane. II. Title.
RJ245.B495 2008
618.92'00231—dc22
            2007060098

Publisher: Julie Levin Alexander
Assistant to Publisher: Regina Bruno
Editor-in-Chief: Maura Connor
Executive Acquisitions Editor: Pamela Lappies
Associate Editor: Michael Giacobbe
Development Editor: Kim Wyatt
Managing Development Editor: Marilyn Meserve
Managing Production Editor: Patrick Walsh
Production Liaison: Anne Garcia
Production Editor: Amy Gehl, Carlisle Editorial Services
Manufacturing Manager: Ilene Sanford
Manufacturing Buyer: Pat Brown
Senior Design Coordinator: Maria Guglielmo
Interior Designer: Wanda España
Cover Designer: Wanda España
Senior Marketing Manager: Frank Del Castillo
Marketing Coordinator: Michael Sirinides
Composition: Carlisle Publishing Services
Cover Printer: Phoenix Color Corporation
Printing and Binding: Courier Kendallville

Notice: Care has been taken to confirm the accuracy of information presented in this book. The authors, editors, and the publisher, however, cannot accept any responsibility for errors or omissions or for consequences from application of the information in this book and make no warranty, express or implied, with respect to its contents.

The authors and publisher have exerted every effort to ensure that drug selections and dosages set forth in this text are in accord with current recommendations and practice at time of publication. However, in view of ongoing research, changes in government regulations, and the constant flow of information relating to drug therapy and drug reactions, the reader is urged to check the package inserts of all drugs for any change in indications of dosage and for added warnings and precautions. This is particularly important when the recommended agent is a new and/or infrequently employed drug.

Pearson Education, Ltd.
Pearson Education Australia Pty., Limited
Pearson Education Singapore, Pte. Ltd.
Pearson Education North Asia Ltd.
Pearson Education Canada Ltd.

Pearson Educación de Mexico, S.A. de C.V.
Pearson Education—Japan
Pearson Education Malaysia, Pte. Ltd.
Pearson Education, Upper Saddle River, New Jersey

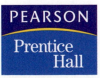

10 9 8 7 6 5 4 3 2 1
ISBN-13: 978-0-13-613554-8
ISBN-10:   0-13-613554-4

Contents

CHAPTER 9

Intravenous Access 82

CHAPTER 10

Pain Assessment and Management 96

CHAPTER 11

Cardiorespiratory Care 104

Preface

Performance of clinical skills in a safe and competent manner is an important component of nursing interventions. This clinical skills manual is designed to assist you in planning and performing nursing skills. It is both an independent skills procedure manual and an accompaniment to *Pediatric Nursing* and *Child Health Nursing* texts. It is portable so that it can be carried to clinical settings and referred to quickly when you need to perform a skill. As a text companion, it helps you to translate theoretical concepts into performance in caring for health clients in a variety of settings. The book is compact so that it can easily be used by students and nurses in the clinical area.

Skills can be challenging to perform on children because of their differing levels of growth and development, lack of ability to communicate or understand information about procedures, and some differences from techniques in adults. This clinical skills manual is intended to enable practitioners to assist in and safely carry out skills commonly performed on newborns and children.

Skills are grouped into chapters that reflect types of intervention. The following chapters are included:

- Protective methods
- Informed consent for children
- Newborn
- Positioning and restraining therapies
- Transporting the child
- Physical assessment of newborns and children
- Specimen collection
- Administration of medication and irrigation
- Intravenous access for newborns and children
- Pain assessment and management
- Cardiorespiratory care of newborns and children
- Nutrition skills for newborns and children
- Elimination skills for newborns and children
- Skin and musculoskeletal care

Each skill begins with a short description, followed by the preparation needed, equipment and supplies required, and the procedure itself. Rationale is inserted within the presentations to explain the reason for certain preparations and actions. Be sure to read the introduction on the following pages, which lists general guidelines that must be applied whenever performing skills.

The skills are presented concisely to emphasize essential information. This manual builds on the basic skills content in nursing programs; it does not seek to replace a nursing foundations course. Rather, it is designed to emphasize pediatric variations and the essential information needed to perform the most essential skills on newborns, children, and youth. Several approaches are used to assist the student in understanding and carrying out the skills. Photographs provide a visual image of equipment and technique. Margin boxes and tables highlight important safety issues, growth and development considerations, teaching for families, and clinical tips. Students using an accompanying textbook will find icons inserted in the text that indicate when a skill has been described in the skills manual. The student can thus move between these two resources to apply theoretical knowledge readily in the clinical setting. The practicing nurse will likewise find both resources helpful in clinical settings.

The clinical skills manual ends with appendices that provide information on growth grids, blood measure values, and calculation of body surface area for medication administration.

NOTE: Students and nurses should always consult their hospital or institution procedure manual or other references for more detailed and specific information when needed.

Acknowledgments

This clinical skills manual has become a reality through the dedication and hard work of many individuals. First we would like to acknowledge the vision of Maura Connor, our editor-in-chief at Prentice Hall Health, and Pamela Lappies, our acquisitions editor. Both of these visionary women know the importance of clinical skills for student and practicing nurses, and support the provision of this reference manual.

The present edition had contributions and reviews from talented and experienced nurses and educators. Without them we could not have accomplished this revision in a manner that best reflects the current knowledge and practice standards. We wish to thank:

Jenny Clapp, RN, MSN
Clinical Assistant Professor, The University of North
    Carolina at Greensboro
Greensboro, North Carolina

Kay J. Cowan, RNC, MSN
Clinical Associate Professor, The University of North
    Carolina at Greensboro School of Nursing
Greensboro, North Carolina

Mary Erickson, RN, PNP, MPH
Pediatric Division APRN/Nurse Planner, Children's
    Hospitals and Clinics of Minnesota
Minneapolis, Minnesota

Sheryl Scheer Sandahl, MPH, RN, CNP, IBCLC
Assistant Professor, College of St. Scholastica
Duluth, Minnesota

Mary Terhaar, DNSc, RN
Clinical Instructor, Johns Hopkins University
Baltimore, Maryland

Many of the photographs were taken by George Dodson and Roy Ramsey; both of these talented individuals are sensitive to issues related to children and families in clinical settings and are creative and proficient in capturing the images of family members and nurses. We acknowledge as well the contributions of individuals to past editions of the pediatric skills in this manual. Marcia Wellington, Jane Novoa, Karen Frank, and Neysa Dobson assisted by providing material and feedback for prior editions.

Ruth C. Bindler
Jane W. Ball

Introduction

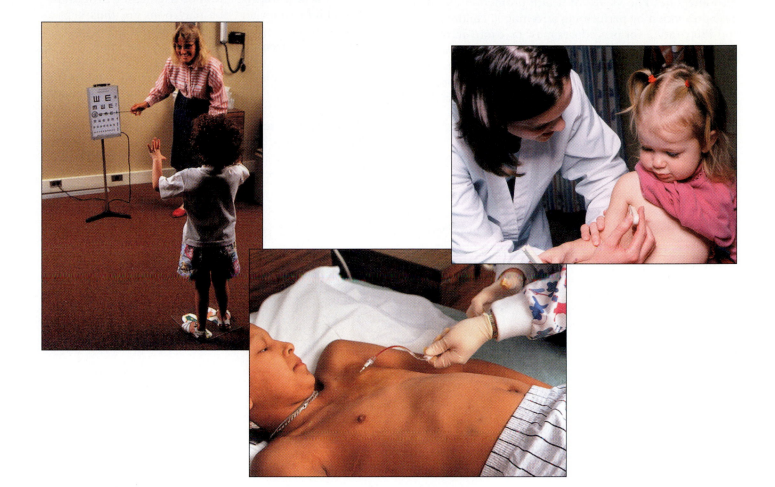

General Guidelines

When a clinical skill is to be performed, general guidelines for performing the procedure include the following:

- Check the medical order to verify the procedure.
- Identify the individual by two types of identification such as name band, medication record, verbal statement, or other means.
- Verify that the consent is signed if needed.
- Greet the individual receiving care and the family members.
- Give developmentally and culturally appropriate explanations and instructions about the specific plan to the individual and family. Arrange for translators to perform the explanation if needed.
- Perform hand hygiene.
- Prepare necessary equipment.

- Don clean or sterile gloves as needed.
- Perform the procedure.
- Clean the area as needed.
- Document the performance of the procedure, results, and responses of the client and family.

Two major concerns the nurse should keep in mind when performing procedures are safety and comfort. The nurse ensures that correct procedures are followed so that the child cared for is kept free from harm. Approaches should be used to promote understanding and comfort for both the child and family members. Nurses play a vital role in skill performance that enhances effectiveness of preventive measures, diagnosis, and treatment in many settings.

Nurses often perform procedures on children in homes, clinics, and hospitals. These procedures, although similar to those performed on adults, differ in several ways. Nurses must therefore be knowledgeable about skills common in child health settings, as well as understanding variations in preparation, equipment, and techniques needed to perform skills on children. The nurse also integrates knowledge of health promotion and disease prevention by performing screening in children.

Preparation for procedures must take into account a child's developmental stage and cognitive ability. Cultural variations may influence how the family perceives the procedures or the language that needs to be used for explanations. General guidelines for preparing the child and family are outlined below.

- Review the technique as needed.

- Explain the procedure to the child and family in a manner they can understand.

- Verify understanding and ask if they have questions about the procedure.

- Inquire if the parent wishes to be present and if the child (when old enough) wants the parent present. If so, clarify the parental role such as immobilizing the child or offering comfort measures.

- Obtain consent for the procedure if needed.

- Obtain necessary equipment and supplies.

Children are taken to a treatment room or to another room for potentially painful or frightening procedures. The child's room and the playroom are thus kept as "safe" areas in which painful procedures are not performed. If parents wish to be present, they can be helped to support the child. When possible, it is best to have other personnel immobilize the child or assist with the procedure so that the child does not view the parent as causing the discomfort. The child and family should receive support after the procedure as needed. Nursing skills provide a unique opportunity to provide a high level of care for parents, children, and families, and to communicate in a sensitive and effective manner.

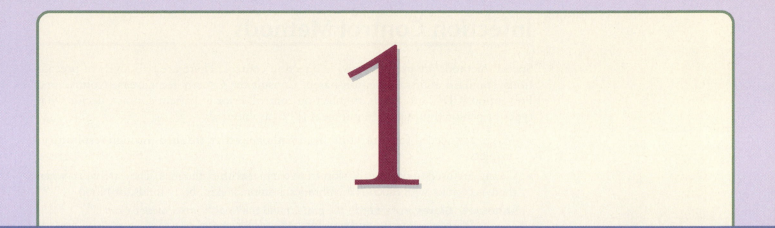

1

Protective Methods

CHAPTER OUTLINE

Infection Control Methods

Infection Control Methods

Special methods are used to provide infection control. There are two levels of precautions: standard and transmission-based. Consult the Centers for Disease Control and Prevention (CDC) for details on infection control. Prior to patient contact, decide what types of personal protective equipment (PPE) are needed:

- *Masks* are needed for protection from pathogens that are shed through respiratory droplets.
- *Gloves* are used to protect the skin from contact with pathogens. They are worn when there is contact with mucous membranes, nonintact skin, body fluids, or blood.

  RATIONALE: *Gloves protect both the patient and the healthcare provider from contamination and transferal of infective agents.*

- *Gowns (protective apparel)* are used for protection against contact with pathogens when it is likely that body substances will come in contact with the healthcare provider's clothing. They are changed before contacts with other patients.
- *Protective eyewear*, such as goggles or face shields, is worn if there is a risk of blood or body fluids being splattered. Wear protective eyewear when the eye, nose, or mouth may be splashed by the patient's body substances and when in close proximity to any open skin lesions.

Standard Precautions

Standard precautions are used in the care of all patients, no matter what their diagnoses, whenever contact with blood, body fluids, secretions, excretions, nonintact skin, mucous membranes, or materials contaminated with these substances might occur. Always have access to protective equipment and add items as needed. The following general guidelines should be used:

1. Conduct hand hygiene before and after patient contact and whenever needed during contact. Wash before donning gloves and after their removal. Soap and water is recommended. Alcohol-based hand rubs are satisfactory when known or visible contaminants are not present (Boyce & Pittet, 2002).
2. Wear gloves whenever contact with blood, body fluids, secretions, excretions, nonintact skin, or mucous membranes might occur. Change gloves each time they are contaminated with these substances, washing hands before regloving.
3. Wear additional protective equipment such as a gown, mask, and goggles if body fluid splashes can occur.
4. Wear the protective equipment listed in this chapter to clean up body fluid spills. Discard waste in appropriate body substance waste containers. Clean the area with bleach or another acceptable cleaner. Bag contaminated laundry in secured and labeled bags.
5. Discard needles, scalpels, and lancets in labeled sharps containers without recapping.
6. Place patients who could contaminate the environment with airborne or droplet infection in private rooms.

Transmission-Based Precautions

In addition to standard precautions, further measures are followed when a patient may be infected with a pathogen or communicable disease. The type of precaution taken is indicated by posting the appropriate sign on the door (Figure 1-1).

There are three levels of transmission-based precautions:

1. Use *airborne precautions* for diseases transported by the airborne route (see Table 1-1). Care providers use high-efficiency particulate air filter respirators (such as a National Institute for Occupational Safety and Health [NIOSH]-certified

STOP: AIRBORNE ISOLATION

VISITORS: REPORT TO NURSE BEFORE ENTERING.

1. Keep room door closed and patient in room.

2. Respiratory Protection.
   Employees wear respirator when entering the room.

3. Use surgical mask on patient during transport.

DROPLET PRECAUTIONS

VISITORS: REPORT TO NURSE BEFORE ENTERING.

1. Wear surgical mask and eye protection when working within 3 feet of patient.

2. Use surgical mask on patient during transport.

CONTACT PRECAUTIONS

VISITORS: REPORT TO NURSE BEFORE ENTERING.

1. Wear personal protective equipment when exposure anticipated (gloves, gowns, mask, and/or eye protection).

2. Use antimicrobial soap for handwashing.

3. After glove removal and handwashing, ensure that hands do not touch potentially contaminated environmental surfaces or items in the patient's room to avoid transfer of microorganisms to other patients or environments.

4. During patient transport drape vehicle with a clean sheet if drainage cannot be contained.

5. Leave routine patient-care equipment in room (examples: BP cuff, stethoscope, thermometer, commode). Clean & disinfect patient-care equipment before use with another patient.

AIRBORNE ISOLATION PRECAUTIONS

VISITORS: PERSONS NOT IMMUNE TO CHICKENPOX OR MEASLES REPORT TO NURSE.

1. Keep room door closed and patient in room.

2. Persons not immune to chickenpox or measles should not enter room.

3. Use surgical mask on patient during transport.

Figure 1-1 *Isolation signs.*

TABLE 1-1	Examples of Diseases Requiring Transmission-Based Precautions	
Airborne	**Droplet**	**Contact**
Measles	*Haemophilus influenzae* type b	Gastrointestinal illness, e.g.
Varicella	Rubella	*Clostridium difficile*
(chickenpox)		*Escherichia coli*
Tuberculosis	Pertussis	Hepatitis A
	Mumps	Skin infections, e.g.
	Pneumonia	Scabies
	Influenza	Impetigo
	Streptococcal pharyngitis	Lice
	Mycoplasma pneumoniae	Genital
		Herpes simplex
		Chlamydia
		Syphilis
		Gonorrhea
		General
		Conjunctivitis
		Methicillin-resistant *Staphylococcus aureus* (MRSA)

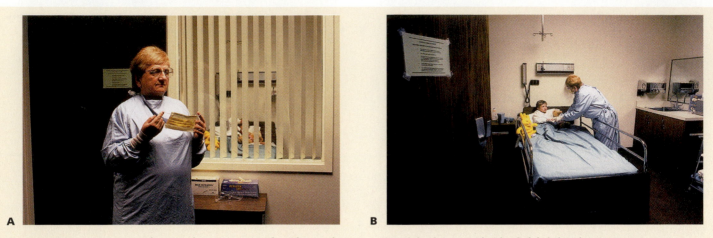

Figure 1-2 *For patients in airborne isolation, gowns and masks may be worn (A), and the door must be clearly labeled with a sign instructing visitors to stop at the nurses' station before entering (B).*

disposable N95 respirator or personal air-purifying respirator [PAPR] hoods and power packs) for protection. In addition, a negative airflow ventilation system room is needed for tuberculosis. The patient in airborne precautions must wear a surgical mask when leaving the room to filter expired air. Label the patient's door with a sign instructing visitors to report to the nurses' desk before entering (Figure 1-2).

2. Institute *droplet precautions* for diseases transmitted by the droplet route. A surgical mask is needed when coming within 3 feet of the patient. The patient wears a mask when leaving the room. The room door can remain open, and special respirators are not required.

   RATIONALE: *The large particle droplets of these diseases cannot travel over 3 feet.*

3. Use *contact precautions* for diseases that spread by direct contact with the skin or by indirect contact with a contaminated object in the patient's environment. Apply gloves for all care. Gowns are worn if the healthcare professional's clothing may come in contact with contaminated surfaces or the patient. Patients should be placed in a private room or with other patients with the same pathogen.

Note: A combination of precautions may be needed. For example, for severe acute respiratory syndrome (SARS), a combination of standard, contact, and airborne precautions must be followed.

> **CLINICAL TIP**
>
> Always use nonlatex gloves if the child has an allergy or sensitivity to latex, or if the healthcare provider has latex sensitivity. See your textbook for information on latex allergy.

SKILL 1-1 Latex Precautions

Latex sensitivity and allergy are antigen-antibody (IgE) reactions to natural rubber latex products. Precautions are needed to ensure that patients and employees with sensitivity and allergy do not come into contact with latex.

PREPARATION

1. Reduce and/or eliminate the amount of latex used in agencies by eliminating use of latex gloves where feasible as well as reducing the amount of other latex products used; when latex gloves are used, they should be nonpowdered.

   RATIONALE: *Powder in latex gloves contains latex which is spread into the environment when the gloves are donned.*

2. Identify latex-free materials and supplies in the agency.

3. Be aware of signs of latex sensitivity.

4. Assess all patients for a history of latex allergy or significant risk factors.

5. Be prepared for emergency resuscitation if needed.

EQUIPMENT AND SUPPLIES

- Latex-free gloves, syringes, and IV ports on IV bags/lines
- Latex-free bellows on ventilator
- Latex-free bags on masks
- Stockinette and latex-free tape
- Medications and equipment for treatment of anaphylactic reaction

PROCEDURE

When patients are identified as latex sensitive or allergic, prepare the environment before their entry and continue practices as long as they remain:

1. Remove all latex-containing products (gloves, tourniquets, tape, etc.) from the room. If latex products cannot be removed, the items should be located in a closed storage area, such as cabinets and drawers.

2. After removing latex items, thoroughly clean the room/exam area using latex-free (nitrile or vinyl) gloves to remove contaminated latex-containing dust. Do not wear latex or rubber gloves to clean the room. When an allergic individual has surgery or other procedure, the room should be properly prepared and the case should be the first of the day.

3. Mattresses/exam tables may contain latex and should be covered completely with a nonlatex protective cover.

4. Stock rooms with latex-free materials and latex-free gloves.

5. Place a latex precaution sign on the patient's door/exam area.

6. Place all monitoring devices and cords/tubes (oximeter, blood pressure, electrocardiograph wires, ports on intravenous tubing) in stockinette, and tape with nonlatex tape to prevent direct skin contact. Items sterilized in ethylene oxide must be rinsed before use. Residual ethylene oxide can cause an allergic response in a latex-allergic patient.

7. Use stopcocks to inject drugs rather than latex ports.

8. Label the patient's medical record, medication form, and identification bands with allergy alerts.

9. Document measures taken.

10. Report promptly and document any signs of sensitivity or allergy.

11. Teach patients and families about latex allergy and how to avoid latex products.

12. Instruct the family about foods that commonly cause allergies in those with latex allergy, and avoid feeding them to the patient. They include bananas, avocados, kiwis, plums, peaches, cherries, apricots, figs, papayas, tomatoes, potatoes, and chestnuts.

SKILL 1-2 Visitor Identification and Health Insurance Portability and Accountability Act (HIPAA)

Nurses must reliably identify patients, family members, and other healthcare professionals, and at the same time protect the privacy of patients. The Health Insurance Portability and Accountability Act of 1996 (HIPAA) identifies protected health information (PHI) by establishing standards for the exchange of health information, security standards, and privacy standards. PHI identifies an individual or could reasonably be used to identify an individual. It includes the following information about the patient:

- Name
- Mental or physical condition
- Diagnosis
- Birth, admission, discharge dates
- Social security number
- Insurance or payment information
- Address
- Relatives
- Telephone and fax numbers
- Certification/license numbers

- Vehicle identifiers such as license plate and serial numbers
- Device identifiers and serial numbers
- E-mail address, Web universal resource locator (URL), Internet protocol (IP) address
- Medical record, account and health plan numbers
- Biometric readings such as fingerprints
- Full face photographic images and any comparable images

An organization may not use or disclose protected health information, except as permitted or required by the HIPAA Privacy Rule. Depending on the situation, a patient may or may not need to authorize the use of PHI. A patient does not need to authorize the use or disclosure of PHI in relation to treatment, payment for care, and healthcare operations.

PREPARATION

1. Be knowledgeable about HIPAA regulations.
2. Review organization policies about patient confidentiality.
3. Review organizational safeguards to assist in protection of patient information.
4. Identify the HIPAA officer at the agency of employment.
5. Assess the patient and family's developmental, cognitive, and cultural abilities to understand protected personal health information.
6. Ensure families have received information about their HIPAA rights.
7. Discuss your professional responsibility to ensure information is being shared only with the legally eligible family or care providers.
8. Explain that you will be clarifying the relationship to the patient of all visitors and sharing only appropriate information.
9. Ask the family to identify any anticipated privacy concerns with potential visitors.

EQUIPMENT AND SUPPLIES

- Patient and family name tags, bracelets, or identification badges to be worn while in the agency
- Employee name tag with job position
- Agency description of HIPAA regulations

PROCEDURE

1. Apply identification bracelets immediately upon a person's entry to the healthcare facility.
2. Identify all healthcare providers and visitors and define their relationships to the patient. Verify the identity of a child's parent/guardian for healthcare decisions. If there are family members who are not legally permitted access or decision-making authority for a minor child, note this on the chart.
3. Never allow a patient to be taken off a unit without written permission of the physician and clear identification of the persons involved.
4. Teach the patient and family about HIPAA regulations. Secure the appropriate signatures on HIPAA forms; maintain in the patient's record.
5. Share PHI and treatment information only with the permission of the patient or legal guardian unless it is for ongoing care, payment for treatment, or healthcare operations.
6. Speak in a moderate tone to prevent conversations from being overheard. Lower your voice appropriately in multiple-bed patient rooms, hallways, elevators, and other public places.
7. Do not transmit PHI over nonsecure Internet connections.
8. Secure patient medical records away from public view. Chart in a secure, nonpatient area; use computer screens that time-out quickly when left unattended; and post patient lists or nurse assignments only in staff areas, away from view of the public.
9. Discuss patient care in private areas.
10. Direct other visitors and relatives to the parents for information about the child, the treatments, and the child's condition.
11. Do not unnecessarily discuss patient conditions with colleagues who are not involved in the care.
12. Consult with the agency designee or HIPAA officer when problems or concerns arise.

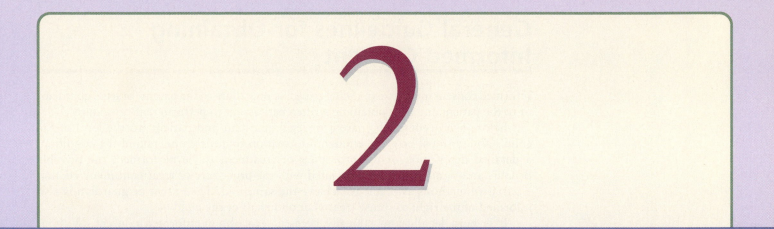

2

Informed Consent

General Guidelines for Obtaining Informed Consent

Informed consent involves explaining a specific procedure to the parent (or legal guardian) or to the patient and then obtaining written permission to perform that procedure.

Before a procedure, the parent or legal guardian and patient (to the level of the child's ability) must be given enough information to clearly understand the condition, a detailed description of the procedure or treatment to be performed, the possible benefits and significant risks associated with the procedure or treatment involved, and alternative methods available to achieve the same end. The parent or guardian is also informed of the right to refuse treatment on behalf of the child.

It is both legally and ethically necessary to obtain informed consent. Without signed permission for medical management, the physician, nurse, or other healthcare provider could be found guilty of assault and battery.

Guidelines have been established to ensure that informed consent is obtained for medical care:

- Information must be presented to the individual responsible for making an informed decision to allow him or her to weigh the benefits of the proposed treatment or procedure against the potential for complications. This information should be presented in simple, easy-to-understand terms. All questions and concerns should be answered honestly and completely.

- The person making a healthcare decision must be over the age of majority (i.e., the age at which full civil rights are accorded—18 years in most states) and must be competent (i.e., he or she must be able to make a decision based on the information received). The person needs to understand the proposed medical management and any risks. In some states, adolescents between the ages of 13 and 18 years are able to sign for some treatment alone (i.e., birth control, substance abuse treatment). Know the parameters of the state law where you practice nursing.

- The decision reached must be voluntary. The person making the decision must not be coerced, forced, under medication that can influence judgment, or placed under duress while considering the options.

Although general written consent for care is obtained within the hospital setting during the admission process, specific consent must be obtained for procedures or treatments that include the following:

- Major surgery
- Minor surgery such as a cutdown, incision and drainage, closed reduction of a fracture, or fracture pinning
- Invasive diagnostic tests such as lumbar puncture, bone marrow aspiration, biopsy, cardiac catheterization, or endoscopy
- Treatments that may involve high risk, such as radiation therapy, chemotherapy, or dialysis
- Any procedure or treatment that falls under the auspices of research
- Photographing patients, even when done for educational purposes

CLINICAL TIP

The Office of Minority Health provides standards related to providing services for clients with limited English proficiency (LEP). They require provision of bilingual staff or interpreter services. Nurses often keep lists of translators and arrange for them to provide services when necessary for children and families. Even if proficient in both languages, children should never be asked to provide translation services regarding healthcare issues due to possible sensitivity and complexity of such data.

SKILL 2-1 Pediatric Considerations for Obtaining Informed Consent

PREPARATION

1. Assess the parent's knowledge about the procedure so that during the discussion with the physician, correct information can be reinforced and misconceptions can be clarified.
2. Assess the child's ability to understand information and participate in the decision-making process.

- If the child is a *minor* (has not reached the age of majority—under the age of 18 years in most states), his or her parent or legal guardian must give consent for all procedures or treatments. Children should become more actively involved in decision making about treatment procedures as their reasoning skills develop. Children too young to give informed consent can be given age-appropriate information about their condition and asked about their care preferences. Their parents, however, make ultimate decisions regarding their care. *Mature minors* (14- and 15-year-old adolescents who are able to understand treatment risks) can give consent for treatment or refuse treatment in some states.

    RATIONALE: *By 7 or 8 years of age, a child is able to understand concrete explanations about informed consent for research participation. By age 11 years, a child's abstract reasoning and logic are advanced. By age 14 years, an adolescent can weigh options and make decisions regarding consent similarly to an adult.*

- Some states provide for the rights of non-emancipated teens to make certain healthcare decisions. The child may give permission only for those conditions identified in state law, and only at the ages specified by that particular state. Some examples of the treatments that many states permit adolescents to sign for include birth control, treatment of sexually transmitted infections, contraceptive and abortion counseling and services, prenatal care, parenting issues, substance abuse, and participation in research (Tillett, 2005). Check the law in your state for specific guidelines.

- If the child is an *emancipated minor* (under the age of 18 years but legally independent from the parents), the child may give informed consent for medical care. Common examples of emancipated minors include teenagers who are married, in the military, living apart from their parents and financially independent, or pregnant or parents themselves. Emancipation is a title given by courts of law, and the adolescent will have a legal document verifying the emancipation.

3. If a parent or guardian is not available, determine that an authorized adult can give informed consent.

    - When a parent or guardian is unavailable to provide consent for treatment, the person responsible for the child (e.g., relative, babysitter, teacher, or camp counselor) may give consent for emergency treatment if the person has signed written permission from the parent/guardian to authorize care in his or her absence. When the parent or guardian can be contacted by telephone, verbal consent can be obtained with two witnesses listening simultaneously. The consent should be recorded for later signature. Under the federal Emergency Medical Treatment and Labor Act (EMTALA), a minor can be examined, treated, stabilized, and even transferred to another hospital for emergency care when the parent or legal guardian is not available to provide consent (for more information, consult http://www.cms.hhs.gov/providers/emtala/default.asp).

EQUIPMENT AND SUPPLIES

- Private area to comply with HIPAA regulations (see Chapter 1)
- Appropriate forms and educational materials
- Pen

PROCEDURE

1. Notify the physician or other healthcare provider that the family is available to discuss the procedure.
2. Obtain necessary forms and written explanations of the procedure.
3. Find a quiet and private place where the physician/provider and nurse can confidentially explain the forms and procedure to the child and/or family.
4. Accompany the physician/provider to serve as a witness and to assist with answering the family's questions.

    RATIONALE: *The nurse's role is to serve as a witness for the physician/provider that the family was fully informed about the procedure and their right to consent to or refuse treatment. The nurse also assists by ensuring that the information provided is understood by the family and put into a context that has meaning to the family.*

5. Ask the family several questions to evaluate their understanding. Provide additional information when any points need to be clarified.
6. When the family appears to have no more questions, ask if they are prepared to give consent for the procedure or need more time to consider their options.
7. When the family is prepared to give consent, the physician/provider and nurse obtain their signatures and serve as witness to their consent.

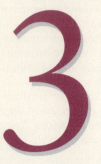

Newborn

Nasal Pharyngeal Suctioning

Immediately following birth, look for mucus in the newborn's nose and mouth and remove it with a bulb syringe as needed. If there is excessive mucus or respiratory distress, suction the newborn with a mucus trap, as described in this procedure.

SKILL 3-1 Performing Nasal Pharyngeal Suctioning

PREPARATION

1. Suction equipment is always available in the birthing area to clear secretions from the newborn's nose or oropharynx if respirations are depressed or if amniotic fluid was meconium stained.

2. Tighten the lid on the DeLee mucus trap or other suction device collection bottle.
   RATIONALE: *This avoids spillage of secretions and prevents air from leaking out of the lid.*

3. Connect one end of the DeLee tubing to low suction.

4. Have blow-by oxygen available to be used with the DeLee mucus trap.

EQUIPMENT AND SUPPLIES

- DeLee mucus trap or other suction device

PROCEDURE *Clean Gloves*

1. Don gloves.

2. Without applying suction, insert the free end of the DeLee tubing 3 to 5 inches into the newborn's nose or mouth (Figure 3-1).
   RATIONALE: *Applying suction while passing the tube would interfere with smooth passage of the tube.*

3. Place your thumb over the suction control and begin to apply suction. Continue to suction as you slowly remove the tube, rotating it slightly.
   RATIONALE: *Suctioning during withdrawal removes fluid and avoids redepositing secretions in the newborn's nasopharynx.*

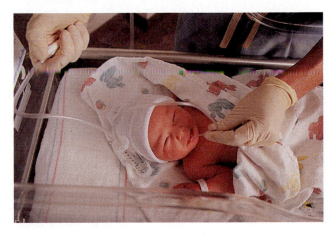

Figure 3-1 *DeLee mucus trap.*

4. Continue to reinsert the tube and provide suction for as long as fluid is aspirated.
   RATIONALE: *Excessive suctioning can cause vagal stimulation, which decreases the heart rate.*

5. If it is necessary to pass the tube into the newborn's stomach to remove meconium secretions that the newborn swallowed before birth, insert the tube through the newborn's mouth into the stomach. Apply suction and continue to suction as you withdraw the tube.
   RATIONALE: *Because the newborn's nares are small and delicate, it is easier and faster to pass the suction tube through the mouth.*

6. Document the completion of the procedure and the amount and type of secretions.
   RATIONALE: *This documentation provides a record of the intervention and the status of the infant at birth.*

Newborn Apgar

The Apgar score is used to evaluate the physical condition of the newborn at birth. The score summarizes the newborn's progress toward independent function specifically in relation to heart rate, respiratory effort, muscle tone, cry, and irritability. A score of 8 to 10 indicates that the newborn is in good condition. If the Apgar score is 7 or below, resuscitative measures may be needed. A score of 3 or less indicates significant distress and need for assistance. Low Apgar scores are used to identify the need for a higher level of care as well as risk for long-term difficulties.

SKILL 3-2 Assigning Newborn Apgar Scores

PREPARATION

1. Identify the person responsible to assign the Apgar score.
2. Preheat the radiant warmer to 36.5°C. (97.5°F)
3. Prewarm blankets under the warmer.

EQUIPMENT AND SUPPLIES

- Apgar timer or digital timer that counts seconds or a timepiece with a second hand
- Infant warmer with ISC and probe preheated
- Clean gloves
- Stethoscope
- Sterile baby blanket

PROCEDURE

1. Don gloves.

   RATIONALE: *A newborn infant is wet with amniotic fluid, vernix, and secretions. Consequently, universal precautions are indicated when handling the newborn until the initial bath is completed.*

> **CLINICAL TIP**
>
> Heart rate and respirations are the two most significant categories to evaluate.

2. Using the following five criteria, determine a score in each and assign an Apgar score at 1 minute.
   - *Heart rate*—Palpate the pulse at the base of the umbilical cord for 6 seconds and multiply by 10, or use the stethoscope to auscultate the heart rate. Score as follows:
     0—no heart rate detected
     1—heart rate below 100
     2—heart rate 100 or higher
   - *Respiratory effort*—Observe respirations and cry. Score as follows:
     0—no respiratory effort or cry
     1—slow to breathe, weak cry
     2—robust cry, good respiratory effort
   - *Muscle tone*—Assess flexion of extremities and quality of muscle tone. Score as follows:
     0—flaccid
     1—some flexion of extremities
     2—active motion
   - *Reflex irritability*—Assess response to noxious stimuli such as vitamin K injection. Score as follows:
     0—no response
     1—grimace
     2—cry
   - *Color*—Assess skin color and score as follows:
     0—generally poor color, pale or cyanotic
     1—body is pink with some pallor or cyanosis over extremities, around mouth or eyes
     2—pink

     RATIONALE: *Assessing these five parameters provides a quick indication of the newborn's adaptation to extrauterine life. With practice, caregivers become skilled at assigning an accurate score. Repeat the score at 5 minutes and again at 10 minutes as indicated.*

3. Document appropriately in the medical record.

Thermoregulation of the Newborn

A neutral thermal environment is essential to minimize the newborn's need for increased oxygen consumption and the use of calories to maintain body heat. If the newborn becomes hypothermic, the body's response can lead to metabolic acidosis, hypoxia, and shock.

SKILL 3-3 Thermoregulation of the Newborn

PREPARATION

1. Prewarm the incubator or radiant warmer. Make sure warm towels and/or lightweight blankets are available.

2. Maintain the temperature of the birthing room at 22°C (71°F), with a relative humidity of 60% to 65%.

   RATIONALE: *The change from a warm, moist intrauterine environment to a cool, dry drafty environment stresses the newborn's immature thermoregulation system.*

EQUIPMENT AND SUPPLIES

- Prewarmed towels or blankets
- Infant stocking cap
- Servocontrol probe
- Infant T-shirt and diaper
- Open crib

PROCEDURE *Clean Gloves*

1. Don gloves.

   RATIONALE: *Gloves are worn whenever there is the possibility of contact with body fluids—in this case, a newborn wet with amniotic fluid, vernix, and maternal blood.*

2. Place the newborn under the radiant warmer. Wipe the newborn free of blood, fluid, and excess vernix, especially from the head, using prewarmed towels.

   RATIONALE: *The radiant warmer creates a heat-gaining environment. Drying is important to prevent the loss of body heat through evaporation.*

3. If the newborn is stable, wrap him or her in a prewarmed blanket, apply a stocking cap, and carry the newborn to the mother. The mother and her support person can hold and enjoy the newborn together. Alternatively, carry the newborn wrapped to the mother, loosen the blanket, and place the infant skin to skin on the mother's chest under a warmed blanket.

   RATIONALE: *Use of a prewarmed blanket reduces convection heat loss and facilitates maternal-newborn contact without compromising the newborn's thermoregulation. Skin-to-skin contact with the mother or father helps maintain the newborn's temperature.*

4. After the newborn has spent time with the parents, return him or her to the radiant warmer. Leave the newborn uncovered (except for the cap and diaper) under the radiant warmer.

   RATIONALE: *Radiant heat warms the outer skin surface, so the skin needs to be exposed.*

5. Tape a servocontrol probe on the newborn's anterior abdominal wall, with the metal side next to the skin. Do not place it over the ribs. Secure the probe with porous tape or a foil-covered aluminum heat deflector patch. Figure 3-2 shows a newborn with a skin probe. Note that in this picture the newborn is no longer wearing a stocking cap.

6. Turn the heater to servocontrol mode so that the abdominal skin is maintained at 36.5°C to 37°C (97.5°F to 98.6°F).

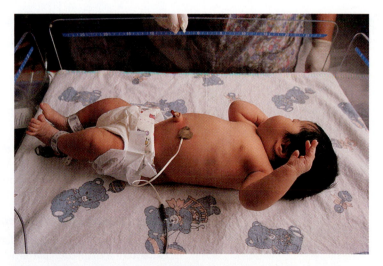

Figure 3-2 *Temperature monitoring for the newborn. A skin thermal sensor is placed on the newborn's abdomen, upper thigh, or arm and secured with porous tape or a foil-covered foam pad.*

Take action to help the new-born maintain a stable tem-perature:

- Keep the newborn's clothing and bedding dry.
- Double-wrap the newborn and put a stocking cap on him or her.
- Use the radiant warmer during procedures.
- Reduce the newborn's exposure to drafts.
- Warm objects that will be in contact with the newborn (e.g., stethoscopes).
- Encourage the mother to snuggle with the newborn under blankets or to breastfeed the newborn with hat and light cover on.

7. Monitor the newborn's axillary and skin probe temperatures per agency protocol.
   RATIONALE: *The temperature indicator on the radiant warmer continually displays the newborn's probe temperature. The axillary temperature is checked to ensure that the machine is accurately recording the newborn's temperature.*

8. When the newborn's temperature reaches 37°C (98.6°F), add a T-shirt, double-wrap the infant (two blankets), and place the newborn in an open crib.

9. Recheck the newborn's temperature in 1 hour and regularly thereafter according to agency policy.
   RATIONALE: *It is important to monitor the newborn's ability to maintain his or her own thermoregulation.*

10. If the newborn's temperature drops below 36.1°C (97°F), rewarm the infant gradually. Place the infant (unclothed except for a diaper) under the radiant warmer with a servocontrol probe on the anterior abdominal wall.
    RATIONALE: *Rapid heating can lead to hyperthermia, which is associated with apnea, insensible water loss, and increased metabolic rate.*

11. Recheck the newborn's temperature in 30 minutes, then hourly.

12. When the temperature reaches 37°C (98.6°F), dress the newborn, remove him or her from the radiant warmer, double-wrap, and place in an open crib. Check the temperature hourly until stable, then regularly according to agency policy.

Umbilical Cord Care

Secure clamping of the umbilical cord is necessary for the transition to extrauterine circulatory patterns and to prevent hemorrhage. Routine care of the umbilical cord helps to promote drying and sloughing of the cord and thus helps to prevent infection.

SKILL 3-4 Umbilical Cord Clamp: Application, Care, and Removal

PREPARATION
1. Obtain necessary supplies.

EQUIPMENT AND SUPPLIES
- Cord clamp
- Prescribed preparations; Triple dye, bacitracin ointment, or isopropyl alcohol for initial cord care
- Cord clamp remover or scissors
- Gloves

PROCEDURE *Cord Clamp Application*
The goal of applying the cord clamp is to prevent bleeding and promote adaptation to the extrauterine circulation pattern.

1. Place a disposable clamp at the base of the cord about 1 inch distal to the skin demarcation line.

2. Secure the clamp by pressing until it clicks and locks.

3. Cut away excess cord distal to the disposable clamp.

4. Examine the cord and count the vessels.

5. Apply agency-specified antimicrobial agent over the base of the cord and on 1 inch of surrounding skin.
   RATIONALE: *Antimicrobial ointments may be used for initial cord care in an attempt to minimize microorganisms and promote drying.*

6. Document status of the clamp and cord in the medical record.

Routine Cord Care

The goal of routine cord care is to promote drying and sloughing of the cord and to prevent infection.

1. Apply diapers so that they are folded below the umbilical cord and do not dampen the cord with urine.

2. Change the diaper frequently to prevent urine from soaking the diaper and cord.

3. Keep the site clean and dry per agency protocol (Figure 3-3).
   RATIONALE: *Wetness and moistness promote growth of microorganisms.*

4. Assess the cord for signs and symptoms of infection (foul smell, redness and drainage, localized heat and tenderness) or bleeding.

5. Document the condition of the cord in the medical record as part of routine assessment.

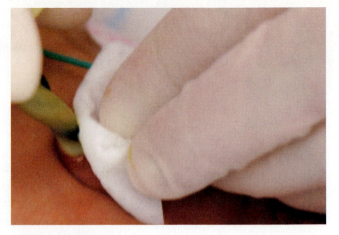

Figure 3-3 *The umbilical cord base is carefully cleaned.*

Cord Clamp Removal

Cord clamps are removed once the site is dry and before discharge.

1. Verify that the stump is thoroughly dry.

2. Apply the cord clamp removal device or insert scissors into the loop at the base of the clamp.

3. Cut through the loop, directing the tool away from the cord and baby.

4. Observe for any oozing or bleeding.

5. Instruct parents regarding care of the site. Advise them to contact their primary care provider if bleeding, oozing, or odor is noticed.

6. Document the condition of the cord and teaching in the medical record.

Circumcision Care

Circumcision is performed on male newborns whose parents elect to have the procedure performed. It is performed once the infant has demonstrated the ability to maintain his own temperature and in most cases prior to discharge.

SKILL 3-5 Assisting with Circumcision and Providing Circumcision Care

PREPARATION

1. Verify that parental consent has been obtained.

2. Medicate the infant for pain.

3. Plan for distraction.

4. Plan for safe positioning.

5. Plan to prevent unnecessary heat loss.

6. Obtain necessary supplies.

7. Coordinate timing to avoid performing the procedure within 3 to 4 hours after feeding.

EQUIPMENT AND SUPPLIES

- Infant warmer
- Circumcision board

- Iodine skin prep
- Circumcision tray
- Analgesia medications
- Pacifier
- Sucrose solution
- Vaseline gauze
- Clean diaper
- Gloves

PROCEDURE *Assisting with Circumcision*

The goal of assisting with circumcision is to provide for the safety of the newborn and to relieve discomfort during the procedure.

1. Check the identity of the newborn, comparing the ID number on the infant bands with the number in the medical record with the circumcision order.
2. Confirm that the newborn has been NPO for 3 hours or as ordered.
3. Have equipment and medications available for medicating the newborn for pain as ordered.
4. Secure the infant to the circumcision board using Velcro straps or other restraint devices.
5. Provide sucrose as ordered for comfort. Offer a pacifier for nonnutritive sucking.

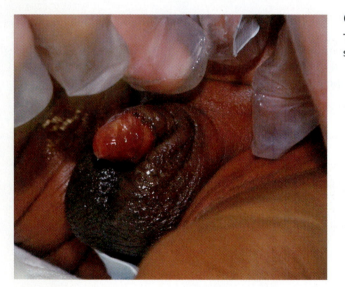

Figure 3-4 *Following circumcision, petroleum jelly may be applied to the site for the next few diaper changes.*

Care Following Circumcision

The goal of care following circumcision is to reduce trauma to the surgical site and to observe for signs of complications.

1. Apply petroleum gauze or jelly to the head of the penis (Figure 3-4).
   RATIONALE: *This prevents the diaper from adhering to the surgical site and reduces trauma.*
2. Apply a clean diaper.
3. Assess the ability to void. Document urination following the procedure in the medical record.
   RATIONALE: *Swelling or injury may obstruct the urethral opening.*
4. Return the newborn to his parents. Explain the procedure.
5. Teach parents to apply petroleum jelly to the site and use A&D ointment to prevent adherence of the diaper to the surgical site.
6. Monitor temperature.
7. Check the site hourly until discharge. Note any bleeding, discharge, temperature, or inability to void in the medical record.

Newborn Bath

At birth the newborn is wet and slippery. The nurse dries the infant under the radiant warmer, wiping away amniotic fluid, blood, and excess vernix using prewarmed towels. The initial bath is generally delayed until the newborn's temperature and other vital signs are stable. Depending upon agency policy and the mother's condition and degree of fatigue, the initial bath may be done by the parents in the birthing room with the nurse's assistance or by the nurse in the nursery.

SKILL 3-6 Initial Newborn Bath

PREPARATION

1. The baby should be resting in a radiant warmer or an incubator.
2. Prewarm all baby blankets to be used.
3. Gather equipment and supplies.

EQUIPMENT AND SUPPLIES

- Clean gloves
- Warm water
- Washcloths
- Blankets or towels for drying

PROCEDURE

1. Assess newborn temperature. Once the newborn has demonstrated the ability to maintain a stable temperature greater than 36.5°C (97.5°F), a first bath can be given.

   RATIONALE: *Temperature instability introduces a threat to newborn adaptation that can lead to serious complications, including respiratory distress, hypoglycemia, and acidosis. Preventing cold stress is an important goal for newborn care.*

2. Bathe the baby under the radiant warmer. If feasible, position the warmer close to a sink for a source of warm water. Alternatively, fill a basin with warm water.

   RATIONALE: *The human newborn cannot maintain his or her temperature independently but requires protection against heat loss in the form of warm, dry blankets and hats, or an external heat source such as the warmth of the mother's body or a warmer.*

3. Using a clean, warm, wet washcloth, clean the eyes, washing from the inner to outer canthus of each eye, moving to a clean portion of the washcloth for each eye.

4. Wash the remainder of the face, cleaning the washcloth after each use.

5. A mild soap may be used for the remainder of the bath. Wash the folds of skin in the neck and axilla. Wash between the fingers and toes.

6. Wash the belly, extremities, and back. Wash the groin and diaper area. Dry the baby after each area is washed.

7. Complete cord care according to agency policy.

8. The hair and scalp can be washed using a mild shampoo, typically at a sink. To do so, wrap the baby in a warm blanket with arms tucked inside the blanket out of the way. Hold the infant in a football hold with head extended over the sink. Use the free, cupped hand to bring water from the faucet to the infant's head. Wet the scalp, apply a small quantity of shampoo, lather, and rinse, again using a cupped hand to bring water to the newborn's head. Dry the head thoroughly and apply a cap. (*Note:* The head may also be shampooed over a basin.)

   RATIONALE: *The infant is wrapped for the shampoo to prevent excessive heat loss. Because significant heat loss can occur through the scalp, it is important to work quickly and to dry the head thoroughly. The cap helps retain heat.*

9. Repeat assessment of temperature. If the temperature is normal and stable, dress the newborn in a shirt, diaper, and cap. Wrap the baby and return to parents in an open crib. If the baby's axillary temperature is below 36.4°C (97.5°F), return the baby to the radiant warmer.

10. Document the bath, any significant findings, and temperature in the medical record.

> **CLINICAL TIP**
>
> Use only a small amount of soap. Excessive soap and lather can be difficult to rinse off.

> **CLINICAL TIP**
>
> Some nurses prefer to begin the bath with the shampoo.

Jaundice/Bilirubin

The most common abnormal physical finding in newborns is jaundice. Jaundice is a yellowish discoloration of the skin and sclera of the eyes that develops from the deposit of the yellow pigment bilirubin in fat tissue. Unchecked, hyperbilirubinemia can have toxic effects on the infant's central nervous system.

Phototherapy

Phototherapy is the exposure of the newborn to high-intensity light. It may be used alone or in conjunction with an exchange transfusion to reduce serum bilirubin levels.

SKILL 3-7 The Infant Receiving Phototherapy

PREPARATION

1. Explain the purpose of phototherapy, the procedure itself (including the need to use eye patches), and possible side effects such as dehydration.

2. Note evidence of jaundice in the skin, sclera, and mucous membranes (in infants with darkly pigmented skin). Be sure that recent serum bilirubin levels are available.

    RATIONALE: *The decision to use phototherapy is based on a careful assessment of the newborn's condition over a period of time. The laboratory results prior to starting therapy serve as a baseline to evaluate the effectiveness of therapy.*

EQUIPMENT AND SUPPLIES

- Bank of phototherapy lights and bilimeter
- Eye patches
- Small scale to weigh diapers

PROCEDURE

1. Obtain vital signs, including the axillary temperature.

    RATIONALE: *This provides baseline data.*

2. Remove all of the infant's clothing except the diaper.

    RATIONALE: *Exposure of the newborn to high-intensity light (a bank of fluorescent lightbulbs or bulbs in the blue-white spectrum) decreases serum bilirubin levels in the skin by aiding biliary excretion of unconjugated bilirubin. Because the tissue absorbs the light, best results are obtained when there is maximum skin surface exposure.*

3. Apply eye coverings (eye patches or a bili mask) to the infant according to agency policy.

    RATIONALE: *Eye coverings are used because it is not known if phototherapy injures delicate eye structures, particularly the retina.*

4. Place the infant in an open crib or isolette (more commonly used in preterm infants and infants who are sicker) about 45 to 50 cm below the bank of phototherapy lights. (See Figure 3-5.) Reposition every 2 hours.

    RATIONALE: *The isolette helps the infant maintain his or her temperature while undressed. Repositioning exposes different areas of skin to the lights, prevents the development of pressure areas on the skin, and varies the stimulation the infant receives.*

5. Monitor vital signs every 4 hours with axillary temperatures.

    RATIONALE: *Temperature assessment is indicated to detect hypothermia or hyperthermia. Deviation in pulse and respirations may indicate developing complications.*

6. Check the lights using a bilimeter to ensure safe effective treatment.

7. Cluster care activities.

8. Discontinue phototherapy and remove eye patches at least once per 8-hour shift. Also discontinue phototherapy and remove patches when feeding the infant and when the parents visit.

    RATIONALE: *Care activities are clustered to help ensure that the newborn has maximum time under the lights. Eye patches are removed to assess for signs of complications such as excessive pressure, discharge, or conjunctivitis. Patches are also removed to provide some social stimulation and to promote parental attachment.*

> **CLINICAL TIP**
>
> If the area of jaundice about the eyes begins to disappear, it is probable that the eye patches are allowing light to enter and better eye protection is needed.

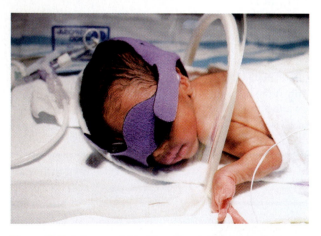

Figure 3-5 *Infant receiving phototherapy. The phototherapy light is positioned over the incubator or crib. Bilateral eye patches are always used during photo light therapy to protect the baby's eyes.*
Source: Courtesy of Lisa Smith-Pedersen, RNC, MSN, NNP.

9. Maintain adequate fluid intake. Evaluate the need for IV fluids.

10. Monitor intake and output carefully. Weigh diapers before discarding. Record quantity and characteristics of each stool.

    RATIONALE: *Infants undergoing phototherapy treatment have increased water loss and loose stools as a result of bilirubin excretion. This increases their risk of dehydration.*

11. Assess specific gravity with each voiding. Weigh the newborn daily.

    RATIONALE: *Specific gravity provides one measure of urine concentration. Highly concentrated urine is associated with a dehydrated state. Weight loss is also a sign of developing dehydration in the newborn.*

12. Observe the infant for signs of perianal excoriation, and institute therapy if it develops.

    RATIONALE: *Perianal excoriation may develop because of the irritating effect of diarrhea stools.*

13. Ensure that serum bilirubin levels are drawn regularly according to orders or agency policy. Turn the phototherapy lights off while the blood is drawn.

    RATIONALE: *Serum bilirubin levels provide the most accurate indication of the effectiveness of phototherapy. They are generally drawn every 12 hours, but at least once daily. The phototherapy lights are turned off to ensure accurate serum bilirubin levels.*

14. Examine the newborn's skin regularly for signs of developing pressure areas, bronzing, maculopapular rash, and changes in degree of jaundice.

    RATIONALE: *Pressure areas may develop if the infant lies in one position for an extended period. A benign, transient bronze discoloration of the skin may occur with phototherapy when the infant has elevated direct serum bilirubin levels or liver disease. A maculopapular rash is another transient side effect of phototherapy that develops occasionally.*

15. Avoid using lotion or ointment on the exposed skin.

    RATIONALE: *Lotion and ointments on a newborn receiving phototherapy may cause skin burns.*

16. Provide parents with opportunities to hold the newborn and assist in the infant's care. Answer their questions accurately and keep them informed of developments or changes.

    RATIONALE: *A sick infant is a source of great anxiety for parents. Information helps them deal with their anxiety. Moreover, they have a right to be kept well informed of their baby's status so that they are able to make informed decisions as needed.*

    NOTE: *Phototherapy may also be provided using lightweight, fiberoptic blankets ("bili blankets"). The baby is wrapped in the blanket, which is plugged into an outlet. The eyes are not covered. With fiberoptic blankets the newborn is readily accessible for care, feedings, and diaper changes. The baby does not get overheated, and fluid and weight loss are not complications of this system. The infant is accessible to the parents, and the procedure seems less alarming to parents than standard phototherapy. A combination of a fiberoptic light source in the mattress under the baby and a standard phototherapy light source above is also used by some agencies. In addition, many agencies and pediatricians use fiberoptic blankets for home care.*

4

Positioning and Restraining Therapies

Guidelines for the use of mechanical and chemical immobilization for children should exist in all healthcare facilities. The Joint Commission on Accreditation of Healthcare Organizations (JCAHO) has specific standards with regard to the use of immobilization, and other organizations set guidelines to assist the healthcare provider. In general these procedures must be prescribed, staff must be trained to use them safely, guidelines for frequency of removal from and assessments should be stated in agency policy, the least restrictive choice for the type of restraint must be made, and they must be used only as long as needed.

Immobilization can be accomplished by holding a child (human restraint), by wrapping with a blanket or other devices (mechanical restraint), or by sedation (chemical restraint). A preferred method of immobilization is to have a trained person be present with a child so that observation can replace mechanical or chemical measures whenever possible. For example, when a child must be held in position for a procedure, it is important to try to use an assistant rather than a mechanical device for this purpose.

Although some parents are comfortable holding their child for a procedure, most prefer to be close and act as a support person and allow health professionals to position and hold the child. This allows the parent to be free to provide comfort and to avoid the role of holding the child for a painful or stressful procedure. The child then can view the parent as a solace rather than as someone who brings pain. With the parent nearby, the child is generally far less anxious and less likely to feel that he or she is being punished. Human and mechanical restraint techniques are described in this section.

BOX 4-1	Recommendations for Restraining Therapies

1. Create the least restrictive but safest environment to maintain dignity and comfort.

2. Use restraining therapies only in clinically appropriate situations and not as a routine component of therapy.

3. Determine if treatment of a condition would decrease the need for restraint. Consider alternatives to use of restraining therapies.

4. Use the least invasive option for restraining therapy to optimize patient safety, comfort, and dignity.

5. Document the rationale for restraint in the patient record. Orders for restraint are limited to 24 hours when their continued need is evaluated and a new order is needed. At least every 8 hours, the potential to discontinue or reduce restraining therapy should be considered.

6. Monitor patients for complications from restraining therapies frequently. Assess every 15 minutes for four times after the first application, and then proceed to every hour as appropriate. Record findings in the patient record.

7. The patient and family should receive ongoing education about the need for and type of restraining therapies.

8. Medications to treat pain and psychiatric disturbance should be used as appropriate to treat conditions and mitigate the need for other restraining therapies, and not overused as a chemical restraint.

9. Use of a chemical restraint requires frequent assessment of actions and side effects. Documentation in the patient record must be performed.

Note: These clinical practice guidelines were developed by the American College of Critical Care Medicine, Society of Critical Care Medicine, and American Association of Critical Care Nurses for maintaining safety in the intensive care unit. However, the principles and guidelines expressed are appropriate for application in all settings. Adapted from Maccioli, Dorman, Brown et al., 2003.

Human Restraint

SKILL 4-1 Positioning a Child for Injections or Intravenous Access

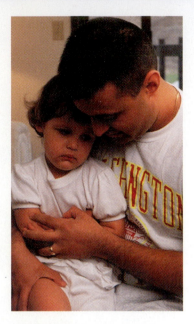

Figure 4-1 *The child should be restrained by the parent or assistant during intramuscular injections. Alternatively to this technique, the child's arm closest to the adult can be wrapped around the adult waist, leaving just the other arm in front to immobilize. Note that the leg not used for the injection is securely located between the adult's legs. Be certain that the child can breathe freely during restraining procedures.*

PREPARATION

1. Determine if the parent wants to be present during an uncomfortable procedure or to be available after the procedure to comfort the child.

2. When the parent wishes to be present, discuss the parent's role (e.g., holding the child or providing distraction or comfort during the procedure).

3. Make sure the person positioning and holding the child (parent or other assistant) clearly understands what body parts must be held still and how to do this safely.

EQUIPMENT AND SUPPLIES

- Supplies for procedure to be performed
- Infection control supplies as needed

PROCEDURE *Supine Position*

1. Place the child in a supine position on a bed or stretcher.
   RATIONALE: *This position allows the child to see what is happening so that some of the child's fear is reduced.*

2. Have the parent, a nurse, or an assistant lean over the child to restrain the child's body and extend the extremity to be used for access or injection.
   RATIONALE: *The nurse's body provides a source of human contact as well as securing the child so that the procedure can be done quickly.*

Sitting Position

Have the child sit on the parent's or assistant's lap with legs held firmly between the assistant's legs. The child's arm closest to the adult can be wrapped around the back of the parent's or assistant's waist.

Have the parent or assistant hold the child firmly against the chest, wrapping arms around the child's upper body (Figure 4-1). Hold firmly but gently, ensuring that the child has chest expansion allowing for normal breathing.

RATIONALE: *This hugging position adds comfort as well as security so the procedure can be done quickly.*

SKILL 4-2 Positioning a Child for Lumbar Puncture

PREPARATION

1. Determine if the parent wants to be present during an uncomfortable procedure or to be available after the procedure to comfort the child.

2. When the parent wishes to be present, discuss the parent's role (e.g., providing distraction or comfort during the procedure).

3. Make sure the person positioning and holding the child clearly understands what body parts must be held still and how to do this safely.

EQUIPMENT AND SUPPLIES

- Supplies for procedure to be performed
- Infection control supplies as needed

PROCEDURE

1. Place the child on his or her side with knees pulled to the abdomen and the neck flexed to the chin. The assistant can hold the child in position by wrapping one arm behind the knees and the other behind the neck, keeping the back curved.
   RATIONALE: *This position ensures the best possible access to spinal processes and disk spaces.*

2. The infant can be held in this position easily by holding the neck and thighs in your hands (Figure 4-2).

3. The older child can be quite strong, and someone with enough strength will be needed to hold him or her in this position. Lean over the child with your entire body, using your forearms against the thighs and around the shoulders and head (Figure 4-3). Alternatively the older child may be in a seated position, bending forward and supported by the assistant.

4. Be certain that the child has free air exchange. Another assistant may be assigned to monitor respirations and perform other assessments during the procedure.

> **NURSING ALERT**
>
> Lumbar puncture requires that the child be held still to prevent injury and to ensure success at obtaining fluid. It is advisable to have an experienced staff member hold the child in position for the procedure. Ensure that the child has free air exchange and receives no injuries.

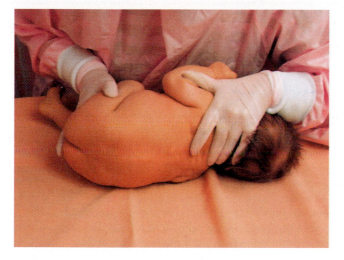

Figure 4-2 *Infant positioned for a lumbar puncture.*

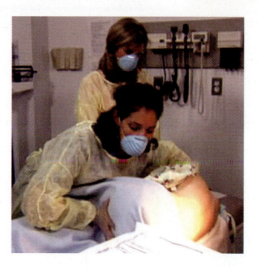

Figure 4-3 *Child positioned for a lumbar puncture.*

SKILL 4-3 Positioning a Child for an Otoscopic Examination

PREPARATION

1. If the parent will be present, discuss the parent's role (e.g., holding the child or providing distraction or comfort during the procedure).

2. Make sure the person positioning and holding the child (parent or other assistant) clearly understands what body parts must be held still and how to do this safely.

EQUIPMENT AND SUPPLIES

- Supplies for procedure to be performed
- Infection control supplies as needed

PROCEDURE *Supine Position*

1. Place the child in a supine position on a bed or stretcher. Have the parent, a nurse, or an assistant lean over the child to position and hold the child's arms and body. The assistant may also assist with stabilizing the child's head.

2. Hold the otoscope in the hand closest to the child's face. When the child is cooperative, rest the back of your hand against the child's head.
   RATIONALE: *This action provides additional stabilization of the child's head to prevent pain and injury when the otoscope earpiece is inserted into the auditory canal.*

3. Use your other hand to pull the pinna toward the back of the head and either up or down (Figure 4-4).
   RATIONALE: *This action straightens the ear canal so that the tympanic membrane can be visualized.*

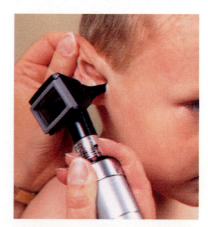

Figure 4-4 *To straighten the auditory canal: pull the pinna back and up for children over 3 years of age; pull the pinna down and back for children under 3 years of age.*

Sitting Position

1. Have the child sit on the parent's or assistant's lap with legs held firmly between the assistant's legs. The child's arms can be wrapped around the parent's or assistant's waist.

2. Have the parent or assistant hold the child's head firmly against the chest with one arm while the other arm holds the arms and upper chest.

   RATIONALE: *This position provides comfort to the child while securing the head.*

Mechanical Restraining Therapies

Temporary mechanical restraining therapies are used to decrease the child's movement and to allow the healthcare provider to carry out a procedure. They are effective when procedures are being performed on the head, or on an extremity as one limb can be left out for the procedure.

SKILL 4-4 Applying a Papoose Board Immobilizer

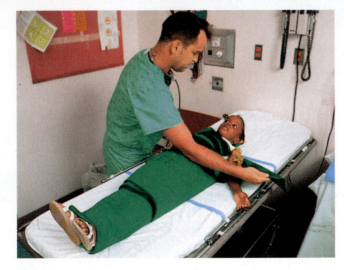

Figure 4-5 *Child on a papoose board.*

The papoose consists of a board and cloth wrappings with Velcro fasteners at the chest, hips, and knees (Figure 4-5). Two sizes are available—one for infants and toddlers and one for larger children. Some papooses come with openings for arms. For example, if the child is positioned for a venipuncture, the arm can fit through the opening in the vest and then the remaining fabric pieces can be secured.

PREPARATION

1. Gather equipment and supplies for the procedure.
   RATIONALE: *Having supplies prepared reduces the time the child spends in temporary restraint devices and reduces the anxiety felt by the child.*

2. Explain the reason for immobilization to the child and parent and how long it will be needed. Tell the child how the restraint will feel.
   RATIONALE: *Young children will be less anxious if the explanation about what they will feel is placed in nonthreatening, developmentally appropriate terms.*

3. Have an assistant (or the parent) available to help position and hold a body part if needed.
   RATIONALE: *The papoose is most often used when the nurse does not have an assistant available or a parent willing to restrain the child for a procedure.*

EQUIPMENT AND SUPPLIES

- Immobilization board (papoose) to fit the child's size
- Sheet
- Infection control supplies as needed

PROCEDURE

1. Place a towel or sheet over the board.

2. Have the child lie supine on the board, with the head at the top.

3. Place the fabric wrappings around the child, and secure the Velcro fasteners. To be most effective, the fabric wrappings should be secure over the elbows, hips, and knees to prevent flexion.
   RATIONALE: *This action prevents the child from pulling apart the wrappings or from kicking.*

4. After the procedure, release the child and allow the parents to provide comfort.

SKILL 4-5 Applying a Mummy Immobilizer

Mummy immobilization consists of wrapping the child securely in a blanket or sheet.

PREPARATION

1. Have all supplies and materials for the procedure collected and ready for use.
2. Explain the procedure to the child and parent.

EQUIPMENT AND SUPPLIES

- Soft blanket or sheet two to three times larger than the child

PROCEDURE

Infant

1. Put the blanket (or sheet) on the bed or examination table. Fold down one corner until it reaches the middle of the blanket.
2. Place the infant in a diagonal position with his or her neck on the folded edge.
3. Bring one side of the blanket over the infant's arm and then under the back. Tuck that edge under and over the other arm and around the back. It may be helpful to roll the infant on the side to smooth the blanket behind the back, and then roll the infant onto the back over the smoothed section of blanket.
4. Bring the other side of the blanket around the body and tuck underneath the body.
5. Bring the bottom corner of the blanket up and over the abdomen.

Toddler and Older Child

1. Put the blanket (or sheet) on the bed or examination table. Fold down one corner until it reaches the middle of the blanket.
2. Place the child on the blanket, positioning so that there is sufficient material to wrap the knees and lower legs. If necessary, fold down the top edges of the blanket to the shoulders.
3. Bring one side of the blanket over the arm, body, and legs, and tuck it under the other arm and around the back and legs (Figure 4-6A).
4. Bring the other side of the blanket up and around the body, and tuck underneath the back and legs (Figure 4-6B and C).

    RATIONALE: *The child should not be able to flex the knees and kick or it may be impossible to perform the procedure.*

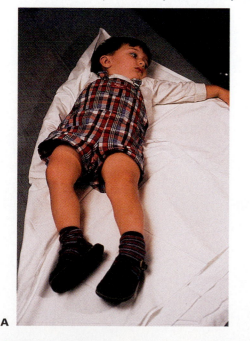 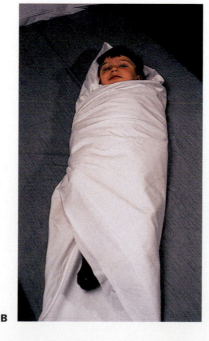 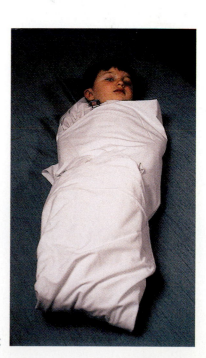

A   B   C

Figure 4-6 *Steps in applying mummy immobilization.*

SKILL 4-6 Applying Elbow Immobilizers

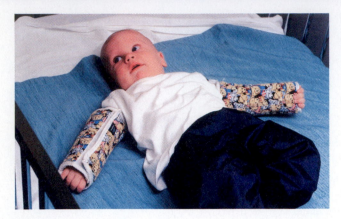

Figure 4-7 *Infant with elbow immobilizers.*

Elbow immobilizers (Figure 4-7) are used to prevent the infant or child from reaching his or her face or head, especially after surgery. Because these devices must be on the child for an extended period, a medical order is required and agency policy is followed for assessments and periodic removal of the devices.

PREPARATION

1. Explain the need for the elbow immobilizers to the parent.
2. Verify the medical order for the device. Review the institution's policy for use of restraining therapies and plan the times when the child is released from them.

EQUIPMENT AND SUPPLIES

- Ready-made elbow immobilizers are available commercially. Obtain them if available.
- An elbow immobilizer can be devised easily from a piece of muslin that has vertical pockets sewn into it. Tongue depressors are inserted into the pockets.
- Pins or tape.

PROCEDURE

1. Wrap the elbow immobilizer around the arm from axilla to wrist snug enough to prevent bending of the elbow.
2. The device may be secured with pins or tape to the bedding or the child's clothing if needed. This type of restraint is more restrictive than just using the immobilizers, should be used only if needed, and requires a written medical order.
3. Remove the elbow immobilizers at least every 2 hours (or the interval specified in the institution's guidelines).
   RATIONALE: *The immobilizer may cause skin abrasion or impair circulation if placed too snugly around the arm.*

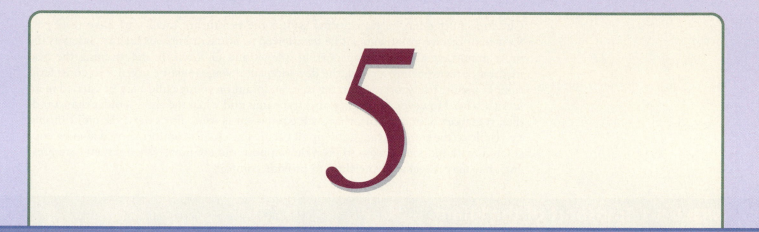

5

Transporting the Child

CHAPTER OUTLINE

Children must often be transported within the healthcare facility to have tests performed or receive treatments, or be transferred to home or another facility. Safety is the most important aspect of transporting infants and children. In determining the best method of transporting a child, the developmental stage must be taken into consideration. For short transports within the unit, an infant or young child may be carried in an adult's arms. However, for transports off the unit and when the child is older than a toddler, transport with cribs or other such equipment is used. For safety, the child should be visible to the transporting adult at all times. The child's comfort should also be considered, with measures taken to promote support and comfort. When parents are present, they may travel with the child to provide comfort.

SKILL 5-1 Transport of the Infant

PREPARATION

1. Obtain necessary transporting equipment.

2. Securely fasten intravenous lines, feeding lines, ECG leads, and other equipment.
   RATIONALE: *Lines that are securely fastened are less likely to be dislodged during transport.*

3. Explain the transport plan to the family.
   RATIONALE: *Adequate explanation helps to decrease anxiety.*

EQUIPMENT AND SUPPLIES

- Transporting vehicle (e.g., stretcher, crib, wheelchair)
- Wheeled poles for any necessary equipment
  - Necessary supportive equipment such as oxygen tank or ventilation bags/masks
- Blankets

PROCEDURE

1. Perform an assessment of the child.
   RATIONALE: *A baseline assessment provides comparison with later findings. At times, transport may adversely affect the child's condition. Initial assessment data provide necessary baseline information.*

2. The infant is placed in a bassinet or crib for transport. If the bassinet has a bottom shelf, it is used for carrying the IV pump or monitor (Figure 5-1).

3. Attach intravenous poles and other equipment to the crib. When this is not possible, adequate personnel are needed to push all of the equipment.
   RATIONALE: *Lines can be more easily kept intact if they are on one transport vehicle.*

4. Keep the infant covered with blankets.
   RATIONALE: *Adequate covers help to prevent hypothermia resulting from a cool environment.*

5. Allow parents to accompany the child on the transport when possible.
   RATIONALE: *The parent's presence can provide a sense of security for the young child.*

SKILL 5-2 Transport of the Toddler

PREPARATION

1. Obtain necessary transporting equipment.

2. Securely fasten intravenous lines, feeding lines, ECG leads, and other equipment.
   RATIONALE: *Lines that are securely fastened are less likely to be dislodged during transport.*

3. Explain the transport plan to the family and child.
   RATIONALE: *Adequate explanation helps to decrease anxiety.*

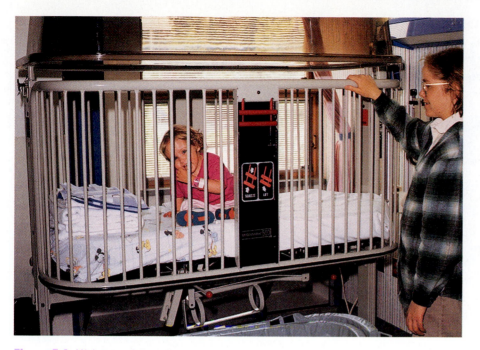

Figure 5-1 *High-top crib for infant or toddler transport.*

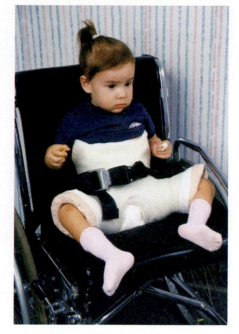

Figure 5-2 *Toddler in a wheelchair with a safety strap.*

EQUIPMENT AND SUPPLIES

- Transporting vehicle (e.g., stretcher, crib, wheelchair) (Figure 5-2)
- Wheeled poles for any necessary equipment
- Necessary supportive equipment such as oxygen tank or ventilation bags/masks
- Blankets

PROCEDURE

1. Transport the toddler in a high-top crib (also used for infants, and shown in Figure 5-1), with the side rails up and the protective top in place. The child may be sitting or lying down. Alternatively, secure the child in a stroller or wheelchair of the proper size for the child's age.

   RATIONALE: *Stretchers should not be used because the mobile toddler may roll or fall off.*

2. Be sure to secure the child in the device with the seat safety strap.

   RATIONALE: *The child is secured to avoid falls and injury during transport.*

> ### CLINICAL TIP
>
> Specialized wheelchairs and other equipment are available to carry enteral feeding solutions, motors necessary for equipment, and other supplies. These transporters are helpful for families when the child has a long-term disability, enabling them to take the child and equipment to school, stores, and other settings.

SKILL 5-3 Transport of the Child with a Disability

PREPARATION

1. Obtain necessary transporting equipment (Figure 5-3).
2. Securely fasten intravenous lines, feeding lines, ECG leads, and other equipment.

   RATIONALE: *Lines that are securely fastened are less likely to be dislodged during transport.*

3. Explain the transport plan to the family and child.

   RATIONALE: *Adequate explanation helps to decrease anxiety.*

EQUIPMENT AND SUPPLIES

- Transporting vehicle (e.g., stretcher, crib, wheelchair)
- Wheeled poles for any necessary equipment
  - Necessary supportive equipment such as oxygen tank or ventilation bags/masks
- Blankets

PROCEDURE

1. Use a wheelchair or stretcher for the older child who is unable to walk because of a disability or whose mobility must be restricted (Figure 5-3).

2. Secure safety belts and supervise the child closely.

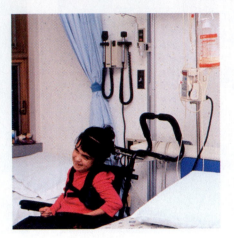

Figure 5-3 *The child who is getting tube feedings or other infusions can easily and safely be transported in a wheelchair with the tube feeding or infusion on a pole. Pumps can also be attached to the pole when used to regulate infusion rates.*

Physical Assessment

Growth Measurements

The accurate assessment of growth is important throughout childhood to ensure the child's health or to identify the impact of disease on the child. Growth charts for boys and girls are provided in Appendix A.

SKILL 6-1 Length

Until a child is 2 years of age, length is measured with the child in the supine position, even after the child is able to stand independently. The length measurement is the standard for accurate assessment of growth in children under 2 years of age. A difference in length and height measurements for children does exist. If height were plotted on a length-based growth chart, a true assessment of the child's growth over time could not be determined.

PREPARATION

1. Have the parent remove any hat or shoes the infant is wearing.

EQUIPMENT AND SUPPLIES

- Measuring board or other length-measuring device

PROCEDURE

1. When using a measuring board, place the infant's head against the top of the board.

2. Use the parent or an assistant to hold the infant's head in the midline, and gently push down on the knees until the legs are straight.
   RATIONALE: *Because of the normally flexed posture of the infant, the body must be extended to obtain an accurate measurement.*

3. Position the heels of the feet on the footboard, and record the length to the nearest 0.5 cm or 1/4 inch (Figure 6-1).

4. Repeat the measurement for accuracy. If a difference between the two readings is found, take the average reading for documentation.

5. Plot the measurement for the child's age on the standardized growth curve. See Appendix A.

If such a measuring device is not available, place the infant on a paper sheet stabilizing the infant in the same manner as when using the board. Make one mark at the vertex of the head and another at the heel. Then measure the distance between the two marks. Record the length in centimeters or inches.

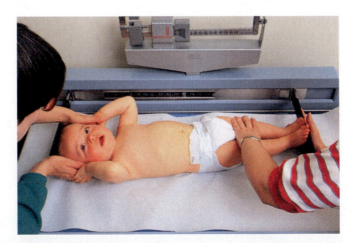

Figure 6-1 *Measuring an infant's length.*

SKILL 6-2 Height

After the age of 2 to 3 years, height is measured with the child standing upright against a wall with a stadiometer (Figure 6-2).

PREPARATION

1. Have the child remove the shoes and hat.

EQUIPMENT AND SUPPLIES

■ Stadiometer or platform scale with stature-measuring device

PROCEDURE

1. With shoes removed, have the child stand straight with the back to the wall. The head should be held erect and in the midline position.

2. The shoulders, buttocks, and heels should touch the wall. The outer canthus of the eyes should be on the same horizontal plane as the external auditory canals.

   RATIONALE: *Positioning the head properly helps ensure consistency in placement of the headpiece on the crown of the head.*

3. Move the headpiece down to touch the crown.

4. Make the height reading to the nearest 0.5 cm or 1/4 inch.

5. Plot the measurement for the child's age on the standardized growth curve. See Appendix A.

In the older child and adolescent, height is often measured using a platform scale with an attached stature-measuring device. Have the child stand erect facing forward. Move the stature-measuring device to the top of the head. Have the child step off the scale, and read the height in centimeters or inches.

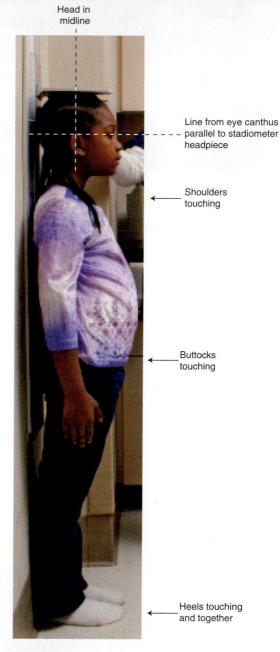

Head in midline

Line from eye canthus parallel to stadiometer headpiece

Shoulders touching

Buttocks touching

Heels touching and together

Figure 6-2 *Measuring a child's height. Position the head in an erect and midline position while the shoulders, buttocks, and heels touch the wall. Move the headpiece down to touch the crown.*

SKILL 6-3 Weight

Infants are weighed on a platform scale (Figure 6-3), in either a supine or sitting position, depending on their age. Take care to ensure the infant's safety. Keep the room warm for comfort.

PREPARATION

1. Check the balance of the scale before using it.

2. Have the parent or assistant remove all of the infant's clothing and diaper. Weigh toddlers in their underclothes. Weigh older children in their street clothes with heavy clothing and shoes removed. Infants with acute diarrheal disease or chronic health problems may need to be weighed nude for accuracy.

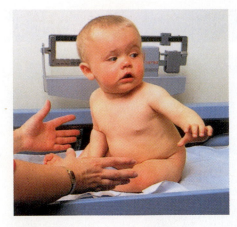

Figure 6-3 *A platform scale is used to weigh an infant.*

CLINICAL TIP

In order to calculate body mass index (BMI), follow these steps:

1. Be sure that weight is in kilograms. If it is in pounds, divide that number by 2.2 to get kg.

2. Change height measurement to meters. Since 1 meter = 39.37 inches (or 0.0254 meters = 1 inch), you need to multiply the child's height in inches by 0.0254 to obtain height in meters.

3. Now square the number of meters.

4. You are ready to calculate BMI. Divide kg of weight by height in meters squared. If a child weighs 26.5 pounds, convert to kg (26.5 pounds = 12 kg). The child's height is 34.5 inches or 0.8763 meters. Then meters² = 0.7679. So the BMI = 15.63.

5. An online BMI calculator is available at http://www.cdc.gov/growthcharts.

RATIONALE: *It is important to try to minimize the amount of clothing worn by children when being weighed to improve comparisons with previous weights taken.*

3. Clean the infant scale tray between uses. Place a paper cover over the scale tray.

EQUIPMENT AND SUPPLIES

- Infant scale for infants
- Paper
- Standing scale for older children

PROCEDURE FOR INFANTS

1. Place the infant on the scale and keep a hand close.
   RATIONALE: *Infants move quickly and it is essential to protect them from falling.*

2. Distract the infant, and take the reading when the infant stops moving.
   RATIONALE: *It takes a few seconds of inactivity for the scale to settle on the infant's actual weight.*

3. Record the weight in the nearest 10 g or 1/2 oz.

4. Plot the measurement for the child's exact age in months on the standardized growth curve. See Appendix A.

PROCEDURE FOR OLDER CHILDREN

The older child can be weighed on a standing scale.

1. Provide privacy for the older child and adolescent.

2. Have the child stand still on the scale.

3. Move the weights until the scale is balanced for the child's weight.

4. Record the weight to the nearest 0.1 kg or 1/4 lb.

SKILL 6-4 Body Mass Index

The body mass index (BMI) uses a formula of kg per m² to assess nutritional status and total body weight relative to height. The child's BMI can be easily determined after plotting the length and weight, or height and weight, on the standardized growth curves. See Appendix A. For more detail, see your textbook.

RATIONALE: *Tracking the change in BMI can often provide clues to nutritional problems, including obesity, health promotion issues, or illness.*

SKILL 6-5 Head Circumference

Head circumference is usually measured at regular intervals until the child's second birthday.

PREPARATION

1. Remove any hat, hair binders, or barrettes the infant is wearing.

EQUIPMENT AND SUPPLIES

- Disposable, nonstretching measuring tape with centimeter and millimeter markings

PROCEDURE

1. Wrap the tape around the head at the supraorbital prominence above the eyebrows, above the ears, and around the occipital prominence (Figure 6-4). Take care to prevent the tape from slipping or causing a paper cut.
   RATIONALE: *This is usually the point of largest circumference of the head.*

2. Record the circumference to the nearest 0.5 cm or 1/8 inch. Repeat the measurement to confirm the reading.

3. Plot the measurement for the child's exact age in months on the standardized growth curve. See Appendix A.

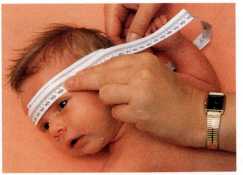

Figure 6-4 *Measuring head circumference.*

SKILL 6-6 Chest Circumference

Chest circumference may be measured until 1 year of age. The chest circumference is a useful measurement in comparison with the head circumference when the growth of either the head or chest is of concern.

PREPARATION

1. Remove all clothing from the child's chest.

EQUIPMENT AND SUPPLIES

- Disposable, nonstretching measuring tape with centimeter and millimeter markings

PROCEDURE

1. Wrap the tape measure around the chest, placed just under the axilla and at the nipple line (Figure 6-5).

2. Record the circumference measurement to the nearest 0.5 cm or 1/8 inch.

3. Compare the chest circumference to the head circumference measurement.

   RATIONALE: *The head and chest circumferences will be approximately equal until after 1 year of age, when the chest circumference begins to surpass head circumference.*

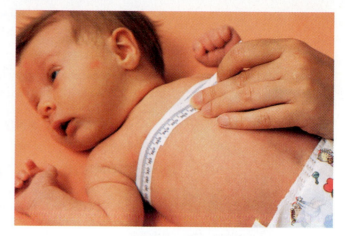

Figure 6-5 *Measuring chest circumference.*

SKILL 6-7 Abdominal Girth

Abdominal girth may occasionally be measured in children to monitor abdominal size that can vary with conditions such as edema from cardiac or renal disease.

PREPARATION

1. Remove all clothing from the abdomen.

EQUIPMENT AND SUPPLIES

- Disposable, nonstretching measuring tape with centimeter and millimeter markings

PROCEDURE

1. Wrap the tape around the abdomen at the level of the umbilicus, taking care to prevent a paper cut.

2. If the measurement is taken at another location on the abdomen, place ink marks at the location of the measurement.

   RATIONALE: *This action will enable you or another nurse to make a future measurement at the same location.*

3. Record the measurement to the nearest 0.5 cm or 1/8 inch. Compare the reading to those taken previously to determine a change in size.

Vital Signs

SKILL 6-8 Heart Rate

The procedure for assessing the heart rate is similar to that for adults. However, an apical heart rate is assessed in infants and young children.

PREPARATION

1. Move clothing away from the anterior chest.
2. Give the infant a pacifier or other distraction to get a resting pulse rate.

EQUIPMENT AND SUPPLIES

- Stethoscope

PROCEDURE

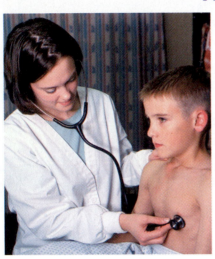

1. Place the cleaned stethoscope on the anterior chest at the fifth intercostal space in a midclavicular position (Figure 6-6).
   RATIONALE: *The apical heart rate is preferred in infants and young children, and it is also used for older children when the condition warrants it. In infants and children, it is difficult to palpate the pulse in an extremity consistently enough to count the rate.*
2. Each "lub-dub" sound is one beat. Count the beats for 1 full minute, or count for 30 seconds and multiply by 2.
3. While auscultating the heart rate, note if the rhythm is regular or irregular. Pulse rates may be palpated in children over 3 years of age. Sites commonly used include the brachial, radial, femoral, and dorsal pedal. In addition, the pulse rhythm, strength, and amplitude may be checked.
   - Note if the rhythm is regular or irregular.
   - Compare the distal and proximal pulses in an extremity for strength.
   - Record if the pulsation is normal, bounding, or thready.

The range of normal heart rates by age is listed in Table 6-1.

Figure 6-6 *Assessing the apical heart rate.*

TABLE 6-1	Normal Heart Rates for Children at Different Ages	
Age	**Heart Rate Range (beats/min)**	**Average Heart Rate (beats/min)**
Newborns	100–170	120
Infants to 2 years	80–130	110
2–6 years	70–120	100
6–10 years	70–110	90
10–16 years	60–100	85

SKILL 6-9 Respiratory Rate

The procedure for measuring a child's respiratory rate is essentially the same as for an adult. However, keep in mind these points:

- Observe the abdomen rather than the chest rise and fall in an infant and young child.
  RATIONALE: *Since an infant's and young child's respirations are diaphragmatic, the abdomen moves more than the chest with breathing.*
- Abdominal movement in a child will be irregular.
- Count breaths for 1 full minute, or count for 30 seconds and multiply by 2.

The range of normal respiratory rates based on age is listed in Table 6-2.

TABLE 6-2	Normal Respiratory Rate Changes for Each Age Group	
Age	**Respiratory Rate per Minute**	
Newborn	30–80	
1 year	20–40	
3 years	20–30	
6 years	16–22	
10 years	16–20	
17 years	12–20	

SKILL 6-10 Blood Pressure

The procedure for blood pressure measurement for the child is basically the same as for an adult. Whether manual or electronic equipment is being used, the correctly sized blood pressure cuff must be selected to obtain an accurate reading (Figure 6-7).

PREPARATION

1. To select the proper cuff size, compare the cuff to the size of the child's upper arm or thigh.

2. The bladder of the cuff should cover about 80% of the circumference of the extremity used.

3. The bladder width should cover about two thirds of the upper arm or thigh.

   RATIONALE: *If the bladder is too small, the blood pressure reading will be falsely high; if it is too large, the pressure will be falsely low.*

EQUIPMENT AND SUPPLIES

- Various sizes blood pressure cuffs
- Electronic blood pressure monitor
- Sphygmomanometer and stethoscope
- A chart of blood pressure values by age, sex, and height percentiles (Appendix B)

PROCEDURE WITH OSCILLOMETRY

Electronic equipment is often used to obtain the systolic blood pressure for infants and young children. With this technique, a transducer uses pressure oscillations received and transmitted by

SAFETY PRECAUTIONS

The American Academy of Pediatrics recommends that sphygmomanometers with mercury columns be replaced by non-mercury blood pressure equipment. If broken, mercury contained in the column could expose healthcare providers and patients to the mercury, a toxic substance. If breakage of equipment with mercury occurs, follow OSHA guidelines for cleaning up the spill.

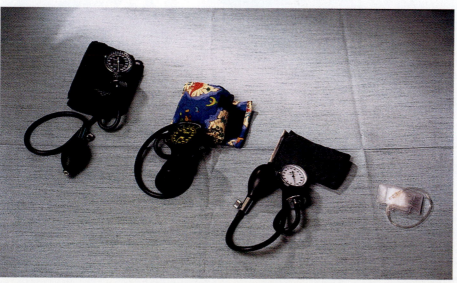

Figure 6-7 *Blood pressure cuffs are available in various types and sizes for pediatric patients.*

CLINICAL TIP

To choose the appropriate cuff size for a newborn, measure the newborn's limb circumference with a measuring tape around the midpoint of the limb used. If the blood pressure cuff has marks to determine fit, use these lines to ensure that the cuff is not too small. The cuff width should not extend to or beyond any joint on the limb used. Make sure the artery mark on the cuff is placed over the brachial artery (Stebor, 2005).

the blood pressure cuff to estimate the blood pressure and mean arterial pressure (Stebor, 2005) (Figure 6-8A).

1. Place the cuff around the desired extremity directly against the skin.
2. Place the arm at heart level with muscles relaxed.
3. Activate the equipment according to the manufacturer's recommendations.
4. Pressure is recorded as the number over "D."
5. Document the blood pressure reading and compare to values for age, sex, and height percentile (Appendix B). Children with a blood pressure reading over the 90th percentile for age, sex, and height percentiles should be referred for evaluation of the elevated blood pressure.

PROCEDURE WITH A MANUAL SPHYGMOMANOMETER

1. Wrap the cuff snugly around the desired extremity directly against the skin.
2. Hold the arm at heart level (Figure 6-8B).
3. Palpate for the pulse, and place the stethoscope over the pulse area.
4. Close the air escape valve. Pump the cuff with the bulb until the gauge rises and no beat is auscultated. Continue pumping until the gauge rises another 20 to 30 mm.
5. Slowly release the air through the valve at 2 to 3 mm/sec while watching the falling gauge.
6. Note the number at which the first return of a pulse is heard; this is the systolic pressure.
7. Continue releasing the air to determine the diastolic pressure: If the child is less than 12 years, a muffled sound will be heard. Record this as the diastolic pressure. If the child is older than 12 years, all sound will disappear at the diastolic pressure.
8. Blood pressure is read as systolic over diastolic pressure (Appendix B).
9. Document the blood pressure reading and compare to values for age, sex, and height percentile (see Appendix B).

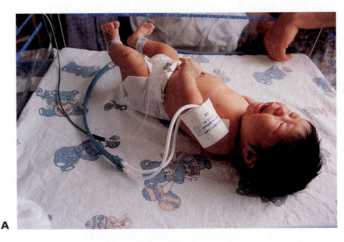

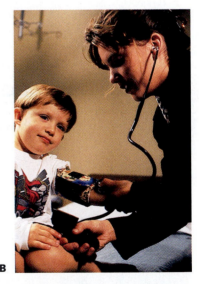

Figure 6-8 *A, Measuring blood pressure using oscillometric technique. B, Measuring blood pressure with a manual cuff. Note the arm is at the same level as the heart.*
A is courtesy of photographer Elena Dorfman.

PROCEDURE FOR BLOOD PRESSURE BY PALPATION

If the pulsation cannot be auscultated, blood pressure can still be measured by palpation. Wrap the cuff around the desired extremity, close the air valve, and palpate for the pulse. Keeping your fingers on the pulse, pump the cuff with the bulb until the pulse is no longer felt. Slowly open the air valve, watching the gauge, and note the number at which the pulse is again palpated. This is the palpated systolic blood pressure, recorded as the number over "P."

Body Temperature

Body temperature can be measured in two scales: fahrenheit or centigrade. Follow the manufacturer's guidelines for the use of electronic thermometers.

The four routes for measuring body temperature are oral, rectal, axillary, and tympanic.

SKILL 6-11 Oral Route

The oral route may be used for the child over 3 years of age who is able to cooperate by holding the thermometer with the mouth closed. The expected temperature is 37°C (98.6°F).

PREPARATION

1. Assess the cooperation of the child to hold the thermometer in the mouth, under the tongue with the mouth closed.

EQUIPMENT AND SUPPLIES

- An electronic nonbreakable probe is preferred.

PROCEDURE

1. Cover the oral probe with the protective sheath.
2. Place the oral probe or an electronic thermometer under the tongue, and have the child close his or her mouth (Figure 6-9).
3. Turn on the scanner and follow the manufacturer's recommendations. It will sound a tone or beep when finished. Remove and dispose of the probe.
4. Read and record the temperature.

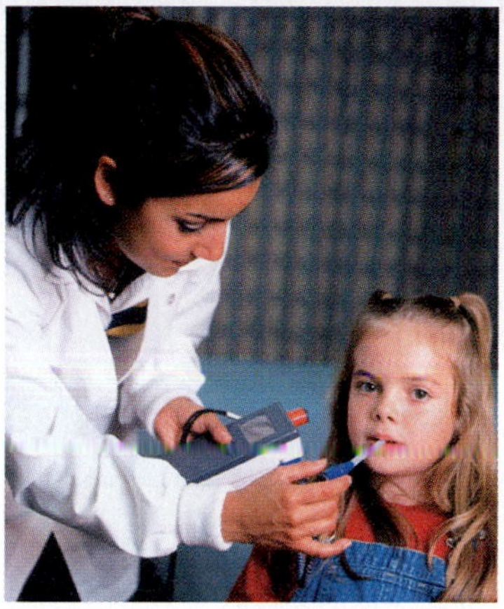

Figure 6-9 *Measuring the oral temperature.*

HOME AND COMMUNITY CARE CONSIDERATIONS

Ask parents what type of thermometer they use at home, and provide instructions in its correct use. They may not know how long to insert the thermometer or how to clean and store it after use. Nurses in schools and childcare centers should assess the knowledge of care providers in these settings and provide teaching as needed.

If the parents still have a mercury thermometer, instruct them to replace it with another type. Some facilities collect mercury thermometers to ensure that they are disposed of properly.

SKILL 6-12 Rectal Route

The rectal route should be used only when no other route is possible, due to the potential for rectal perforation and because most children view this as an intrusive procedure. The rectal temperature is one degree higher than the oral temperature, 37.6°C (99.7°F). The rectal temperature is a close approximation of core body temperature (Craig, Lancaster, Taylor et al., 2002).

PREPARATION

1. Place the infant or child prone on a bed or the parent's lap; turn the older child on the side.

EQUIPMENT AND SUPPLIES

- Electronic thermometer with sheath
- Water-soluble lubricant

PROCEDURE *Clean Gloves*

1. Cover the tip of the electronic thermometer protective sheath with a water-soluble lubricant.
2. For the infant, place the tip 1/4 to 1/2 inch into the rectum. For the child, place the tip 1 inch into the rectum.
   RATIONALE: *This reduces the risk of rectal perforation.*
3. Turn on the scanner and follow the manufacturer's recommendations. It will tone or beep when finished. Remove and dispose of the probe.
4. Read and record the temperature.

SKILL 6-13 Axillary Route

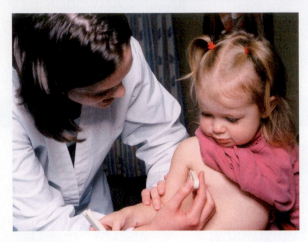

The axillary route is often used for newborns and for children who are seizure-prone, unconscious, or immunosuppressed, or who have a structural abnormality that precludes an alternative route. The axillary temperature is generally 0.6°C (1°F) lower than the oral temperature. Current research indicates that the axillary temperature difference between oral and rectal routes increases when the child's body temperature increases (Falzon, Grech, Caruana et al., 2003). Therefore, the axillary route is not as accurate as other methods for identifying children with fevers.

PROCEDURE

1. The electronic thermometer with protective sheath is held in place in the axilla, with the child's arm pressed close to his or her side (Figure 6-10).

2. Turn on the scanner and follow the manufacturer's recommendations. It will sound a tone or beep when finished. Remove and dispose of the probe.

3. Read and record the temperature.

Figure 6-10 *Measuring the axillary temperature.*

SKILL 6-14 Tympanic Route

The tympanic route is a convenient and fast method for taking temperatures in infants and children. Infrared technology provides a rapid reading. The ear temperature reflects the body temperature because the tympanic membrane shares its blood supply with the hypothalamus. The tympanic thermometer is easy to use, and is noninvasive in nature. However, because of inaccuracies in measurement by this route, the tympanic temperature reading should not be used as an approximation of rectal temperature when a precise reading is important for treatment decisions (Craig, Lancaster, Taylor et al., 2002).

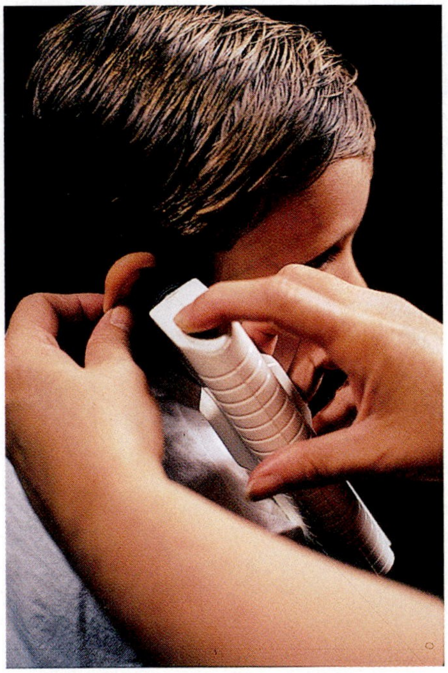

PREPARATION

1. Place the infant in a supine position on a flat surface. Stabilize the infant's head, and turn the infant's head 90 degrees for easy access.

2. Position the child on the parent's or assistant's lap with head secured.

EQUIPMENT AND SUPPLIES

- Tympanic thermometer with clean disposable probe

PROCEDURE *Child Younger than 1 Year*

1. If using the child's right ear, hold the thermometer in your right hand. For the child's left ear, hold the thermometer in your left hand.

2. Pull the pinna of the ear straight back and downward. Approach the ear from behind to direct the tip anteriorly to make sure the thermometer tip is aimed toward the tympanic membrane (Figure 6-11).
   RATIONALE: *The tip must be aimed at the tympanic membrane to ensure accuracy.*

3. Place the probe in the ear as far as possible to seal the canal. Turn on the scanner.

4. Leave the probe in the ear according to the manufacturer's recommendations.

5. Remove the probe, and read and record the temperature.

Child Older than 1 Year

1. Pull the pinna up and back in children over about 3 years or up, and downward under that age.

2. Place the probe and continue as described previously for the child younger than 1 year.

3. Read and record the temperature.

Figure 6-11 *Position for inserting a thermometer when the tympanic route is used. The pinna is pulled up and back to straighten the ear canal in this young child.*

Special Neurologic Assessments

SKILL 6-15 Glasgow Coma Scale

The Glasgow Coma Scale is used to quantify the level of consciousness, thus enabling future comparison of improvement or deterioration in the child's condition. Pediatric criteria, which take into account the child's developmental age for each category of the test, have been established to assess responses to eye opening, verbal response, and motor response (Table 6-3).

PROCEDURE

1. When the child has had an injury to the head or has altered consciousness, assess each of the three categories of the Glasgow Coma Scale according to the criteria in the table.

2. Note the time and score for each category. Total the scores for all three categories to get the Glasgow Coma Score. A score of 15 is the maximum and indicates the best level of neurologic functioning.

3. Repeat the test at regular intervals.
   RATIONALE: *Since the test provides a numeric score for altered consciousness, regular measurements help detect subtle changes in the child's condition.*

4. Document the score and time performed.

TABLE 6-3	Glasgow Coma Scale for Assessment of Coma in Infants and Children	
Category	**Score**	**Infant and Young Child Criteria**
Eye opening	4	Spontaneous opening
	3	To loud noise
	2	To pain
	1	No response
Verbal response	5	Smiles, coos, cries to appropriate stimuli
	4	Irritable; cries
	3	Inappropriate crying
	2	Grunts, moans
	1	No response
Motor response	6	Spontaneous movement
	5	Withdraws to touch
	4	Withdraws to pain
	3	Abnormal flexion (decorticate)
	2	Abnormal extension (decerebrate)
	1	No response

Add the score from each category to get the total. The maximum score is 15, indicating the best level of neurological functioning. The minimum is 3, indicating total neurologic unresponsiveness.

Reprinted from James, H. E. (1986). Neurologic evaluation and support in the child with acute brain insult. *Pediatric Annals, 15*(1), p.17, 1986, with permission from SLACK Incorporated.

SKILL 6-16 Neurovascular Assessment

A neurovascular assessment is performed frequently when an extremity is injured, such as from a fracture or circumferential burn. The circulatory status and nerve function are both evaluated in the injured extremity and compared to the other extremity. See Chapter 14 regarding cast care for a description of this assessment.

PROCEDURE

1. Assess the swelling in the extremity associated with the injury.
   RATIONALE: *The swelling associated with the injury may constrict blood flow to the distal extremity and pinch the nerves, especially when constriction is present, such as a cast.*

2. Assess the extremity distal to the injury for color and temperature and compare to the other extremity.

3. Assess the capillary refill time by pressing on a finger or toe for a couple of seconds, until the skin is blanched. Count how long it takes for blood or color to return to the area pressed. It should take 2 seconds or less.

4. Assess the extremity for pain and sensation (numbness, tingling, pins and needles sensation) and compare to the other extremity.

5. Consider all the findings simultaneously to complete the neurovascular assessment.

6. The presence of most or all of the following indicates significantly impaired circulation and pressure or injury to the nerve that needs emergency intervention:
   - Pallor or cyanosis
   - Capillary refill time greater than 4 seconds
   - Cool or cold temperature
   - Moderate or severe pain
   - Numbness, tingling, or pins and needles sensation

7. Document the assessment, and repeat it frequently, especially if one or two findings are present.
   RATIONALE: *If the circulatory and neurologic constriction is not detected and promptly relieved, permanent damage to the distal extremity may result.*

SKILL 6-17 Intracranial Pressure Monitoring and Daily Care

CLINICAL TIP

Cerebral perfusion pressure (CPP) is calculated by subtracting the ICP from the mean arterial pressure. Normal CPP is 60 to 150 mm Hg. Normal ICP is 5 to 15 mm Hg.

Intracranial pressure (ICP) is the force exerted by brain tissue, cerebrospinal fluid, and the blood within the cranial vault. Increased ICP can result from traumatic brain injury, brain tumors, or infection. Increased intracranial pressure results in decreased cerebral perfusion pressure (CPP) which is the amount of pressure needed to ensure that adequate oxygen and nutrients will be delivered to the brain.

ICP monitoring is often accomplished with intraventricular catheter placement or ventriculostomy. Cerebrospinal fluid (CSF) may also be drained from the ventriculostomy to lower the ICP. Other mechanisms used to monitor the ICP include an intraparenchymal catheter, a subarachnoid/subdural bolt or screw, or an epidural sensor.

PREPARATION

1. Review the patient's chart related to indications for intracranial pressure monitoring.

2. Review the physician's orders for monitoring and drainage parameters.

3. Verify the identity of the child.

4. Assess the child and family's understanding of the need for intracranial pressure monitoring. Provide explanations to the child and family.

EQUIPMENT

ICP transducer system and monitor

PROCEDURE *Sterile Gloves*

1. Assess the system and all connections for leaks and kinked tubing. Maintain the sterility of the equipment.
   RATIONALE: *Patency of the system helps prevent infection and allows for CSF drainage.*

2. Ensure that the fluid-filled transducer system is placed and maintained at the level of the foramen of Monro, the line between the top of the ear and the outer canthus of the eye. Balance the ICP transducer to zero for calibration according to hospital guidelines and when the child's position changes.
   RATIONALE: *This ensures the accuracy of pressure readings and waveforms by the transducer system.*

3. ICP monitoring is usually continuous. Document ICP and CPP at the frequency ordered by the physician or by hospital protocol. Monitor and print ICP waveforms. See Table 6-4.

4. Assess the child's responsiveness, vital signs, and neurologic status. Assess for signs of ICP. See Table 6-5.
   RATIONALE: *Patients with brain injuries are at risk for seizures and cerebral edema, which further compromise CPP.*

TABLE 6-4	ICP Waveforms and Implications	
Waveform	**Pressure mm Hg**	**Implications**
A	50–100	Symptoms related to cerebral dysfunction, changes in vital signs, respiratory pattern, motor function, headache, and emesis
B	20–50	Decreasing level of consciousness, agitation, varying respiratory pattern
C	4–20	No clinical significance
Normal	4–15	Normal

TABLE 6-5	Signs of Increased Intracranial Pressure
Timing of Signs	**Signs**
Early signs	Headache Visual disturbances, diplopia Nausea and vomiting Dizziness or vertigo Slight change in vital signs Pupils not as reactive or equal Sunsetting eyes Seizures Slight change in level of consciousness
Additional signs in infants	Bulging fontanel Wide sutures, increased head circumference Dilated scalp veins High-pitched, catlike cry
Late signs	Significant decrease in level of consciousness Cushing's triad ■ Increased systolic blood pressure and widened pulse pressure ■ Bradycardia ■ Irregular respirations Fixed and dilated pupils

5. Assess pain and comfort level. Administer sedation and pain medication as prescribed.

   RATIONALE: *Patients may experience pain at the catheter insertion site and pain from increased ICP. Medications promote the child's comfort and help reduce elevations in ICP.*

6. Assess the insertion site for bleeding, CSF leakage, and signs and symptoms of infection.

7. If the system is draining CSF, assess the output for color, amount, and quality per unit protocol.

8. Maintain the child's position with the head at midline with the remainder of the body and the head of the bed elevated 15 to 30 degrees.

   RATIONALE: *This position prevents compression of blood vessels in the neck and improves venous blood flow.*

9. Monitor patient neurologic status during nursing care and continue or stop depending on patient response. Document care and patient response.

   RATIONALE: *Some environmental stimuli, the voice, and nursing care procedures may have an effect on ICP and brain compliance (Johnson, 1999). Poor brain compliance is evidenced by: deterioration in clinical signs, increase in ICP greater than 10 mm Hg above baseline longer than 3 minutes, and wide amplitude waveform and/or the appearance of plateau waves.*

10. Document the ICP reading, CPP, waveforms, and the child's neurologic status.

Visual Acuity Screening

Vision acuity screening should begin at about 3 years of age, when the child can cooperate with the procedure. Several procedures may be used to screen visual acuity in children.

SKILL 6-18 Snellen Letter Chart

The Snellen letter (alphabet) chart (Figure 6-12A) is the most commonly used assessment tool for visual acuity. It consists of lines of letters in decreasing size.

- Most charts are designed for reading from a distance of 20 feet. When the child reads the line designated "20 feet" while standing 20 feet away, vision is 20/20. If, however, the child can only read the line labeled "40 feet" while standing 20 feet away, vision is 20/40.
- Charts are also available that can be used at a distance of 10 feet. A child who stands 10 feet from this chart and reads the 10-foot line (10/10) has vision equivalent to that of 20/20 when using the 20-foot chart.

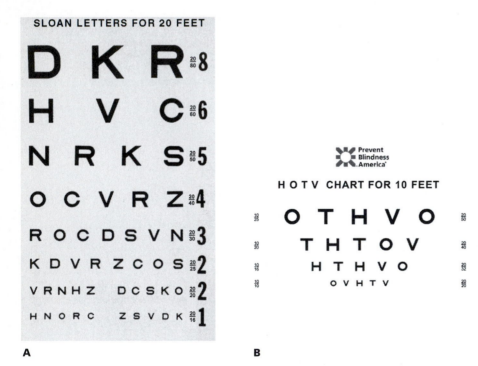

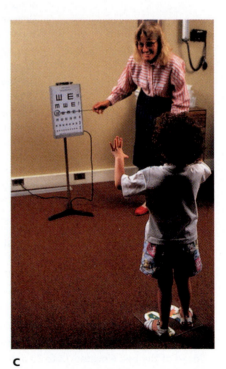

A   B   C

Figure 6-12 *Visual acuity charts. A, Snellen letter chart. B, HOTV chart. C, Snellen E chart.*
A and B courtesy of the National Society for the Prevention of Blindness.

SKILL 6-19 HOTV, Snellen E, or Picture Chart

For toddlers and children who have not yet mastered the alphabet, the HOTV, Snellen E (Figure 6-12B and C), or picture chart may be used, positioned either 10 or 20 feet away.

- The HOTV test uses a chart with the letters H, O, T, and V used in random order on lines in decreasing size. The child either names the letters or points to them on a card held close by. The procedure followed is the same as with the Snellen test, but because children can point to the letters on the chart in front of them, they do not need to know the alphabet. The HOTV test can also be used after a practice session with children who do not speak English.

- In the Snellen E chart, the capital letter E is shown facing in different directions. The child is asked to point in the direction of the "legs" of the E. Another option is to give the child a paper with an E on it and have the child turn it in the direction the E is pointing on the chart.
- The picture chart has commonly identified silhouettes (e.g., house, apple, umbrella). The child is asked to identify the pictures.

PREPARATION

1. The procedure is explained to the child and parent. With a young child, make a game of identifying the letter, direction of the E, or the picture. Practice with the child before starting, providing positive feedback for correct responses.
   RATIONALE: *This ensures that the child understands the directions for the test to improve the chances of an accurate screening test result.*

2. Place the chart at the child's eye level and ensure that it is well lit.

EQUIPMENT AND SUPPLIES

- Screening chart
- Card or other item to cover one eye

PROCEDURE

1. Place the heels of the child at the 20-foot mark (or 10-foot mark if using that chart).

2. Assess each eye separately and then both together. If the child wears glasses, check the vision both with and without glasses. If the child is wearing contacts, leave them in and note that the results were with contacts.
   RATIONALE: *It is important to detect significant differences in visual acuity of the eyes of children under 5 years. When one eye has poorer vision than the other, the brain may decide to stop using the eye with poor vision, leading to further vision deterioration. Corrective lenses are required to enable the child to use both eyes and to preserve vision.*

3. While one eye is being tested, use the child's hand, a patch, or a piece of cardboard to cover the other eye. Tell the child to keep the covered eye open during the testing. Use a different eye cover for each child to minimize the spread of infection among children.

4. Observe for squinting, moving the head forward (to be closer to the chart), excessive blinking, or tearing during the examination.
   RATIONALE: *These may be signs that the child has a vision problem.*

5. Document the last line the child can read correctly (i.e., the last line in which the child reads more than half the symbols on the line). Refer to Table 6-6 for expected visual acuity by age.

6. When a child's vision is not within the passing standards range for age, the child should be retested in 1 to 2 weeks. If the results are still unsatisfactory, make the appropriate referral to the child's pediatrician or other healthcare provider, an ophthalmologist, or an optometrist.

TABLE 6-6	Passing Standards for Visual Acuity Testing Based on Age
Age	**Visual Acuity**
3–4 years	20/40
5 years	20/30
6 years	20/20

Hearing Acuity Screening

It is important to perform hearing acuity screening to ensure that the child is able to hear for speech and language development to occur. Newborn and infant hearing screening is performed using evoked otoacoustic emission and auditory brainstem response. See your textbook for further description of newborn hearing screening.

Several procedures may be used to screen hearing acuity in children. Various conditions during childhood, such as frequent ear infections, could result in a hearing loss.

SKILL 6-20 Pure Tone Audiometry

COMMUNITY CONSIDERATIONS

Each state has specific laws mandating when children attending school should be screened for hearing acuity, and the hertz and decibel levels to be included. Consult your state school code for guidance about local requirements.

This procedure screens for hearing using air conduction. It is used on cooperative children over the age of 3 years. It can detect sensorineural hearing loss, but it does not detect fluid in the middle ear.

PREPARATION

1. When screening a large group of children, such as in a school, the machine may be taken to the classroom for demonstration and practice.
2. Check the transmission of sound to be sure both earphones work properly.
3. Explain the procedure in terms the child can understand. Show the earphones. Turn the sound loud enough for the child to hear and practice raising a hand in response to the sound.
   RATIONALE: *This action helps ensure that accurate results from the screening test are obtained.*
4. If a soundproof room is not available, the audiometer should be set up in a quiet environment.
   RATIONALE: *It is important to reduce exposure to other sources of sound that could interfere with the child's response to the audiometer's sounds.*
5. Clean the earphones with alcohol swabs between children.
   RATIONALE: *This practice removes most microorganisms for infection control between children.*

GROWTH AND DEVELOPMENT

If the young child does not seem to understand what to do once screening begins, remove the headphones and practice more. Have blocks ready and instruct the child to place a block in a basket when hearing the sound. Turn up the decibel level slightly and practice until the child understands. Then turn the decibel level back to the appropriate screening level.

EQUIPMENT AND SUPPLIES

- Calibrated audiometer
- Scoring sheet
- Alcohol swabs

PROCEDURE

1. Position the child so that his or her back is toward the machine and faced away from the tester.
   RATIONALE: *This position ensures that the child cannot see the examiner press the lever to present the sound, and cannot receive visual cues from the examiner's face when the sound is presented.*
2. Place the headset on the child's head and adjust for a proper fit. Note the right and left indicators on the earphones.
3. Follow directions for using the audiometer. Deliver sounds and watch for the child to raise a hand when heard. The sound cue is given to the child using a random order when testing the ears.
   RATIONALE: *This action ensures that the child cannot anticipate the sound and potentially cause an inaccurate interpretation of the screening test.*
4. Test each ear at the following pitches: 500, 1000, 2000, and 4000 Hz at increasing levels of loudness (decibels).
5. If the child does not pass the screening with both ears, retest the child in 2 weeks. If the child still does not pass, refer for further evaluation (Table 6-7).
   RATIONALE: *The child with an upper respiratory infection may not hear well and needs time for the infection to improve. Continued failure of the screening may indicate a hearing problem.*
6. Document the results of the hearing test.

CLINICAL TIP

The sounds of the audiometer are delivered at hertz levels, or the frequency of sound in cycles per second. Lower numbers indicate lower frequency sounds, such as speech tones. Higher numbers indicate higher frequency sounds, such as heard in music. The decibels, loudness of the sounds, can also be controlled by the audiometer.

TABLE 6-7	Passing Standards for Hearing Acuity with Pure Tone Audiometer
Hertz	**Decibels**
500	20–25
1000	20–25
2000	20–25
4000	25

SKILL 6-21 Tympanometry

Tympanometry provides an estimate of middle ear pressure and an indirect measure of tympanic membrane compliance (movement). Older infants and children can be tested. Abnormal findings often indicate fluid accumulation in the middle ear that prevents the efficient transmission of sound to the inner ear. This can result in hearing loss over time.

PREPARATION

1. Explain the procedure to the child and parents and the need for the child to hold still.

EQUIPMENT AND SUPPLIES

- Calibrated tympanometer
- Disposable earpiece
- Graph paper

PROCEDURE

1. Encourage the child to hold still during the test. The infant and young child may need assistance in holding still.
   RATIONALE: *Lack of movement reduces the chance of pain or injury from the earpiece in the auditory canal.*

2. Gently insert the earpiece with the tympanometer probe into the auditory canal until the canal is sealed and airtight.
   RATIONALE: *The canal must be sealed tight to get an accurate measurement of the pressure needed to move the tympanic membrane.*

3. Turn on the tympanometer according to manufacturer instructions and emit the tone. The pressure is measured by the probe and plots it on a graph (Figure 6-13A and B).

4. Repeat the procedure in the other ear.

5. Insert the printout into the child's medical record and document the results of the test.

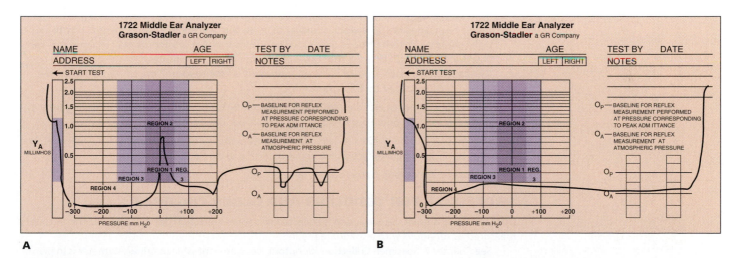

A **B**

Figure 6-13 A, *This tympanogram demonstrates normal hearing as evidenced by the curve showing the tympanic membrane's movement when a sound wave is emitted into the ear canal. Mobility is between 0.2 mL and 1 mL, the normal range. B, In contrast, note the flat pattern in the second tympanogram, which shows very restricted mobility of the tympanic membrane in response to sound.*

Fluid and Electrolyte Balance: Intake and Output

Intake and output (I and O) is a measurement of fluid and electrolyte balance in the body. Input is measured as for adults, recording the fluids delivered to the child through parenteral or oral routes in milliliters (mL). See your textbook for more details.

Output is a measurement of what is expelled, drained, secreted, or suctioned from the body. Output sources include urine, stool, vomitus, sweat, drainage from wounds, and nasogastric suction. Output for older children can be measured as for adults with a graduated cylinder, and recorded in cubic centimeters (cc) or milliliters (mL).

Accurate measurement of I and O is documented for many children, such as those receiving IV fluids or certain medications, after major surgery, and those with serious infections, renal disease or kidney damage, congestive heart failure, diabetes mellitus, dehydration or hypovolemia, or severe thermal burns.

SKILL 6-22 Output Measurement

PREPARATION

1. Weigh the diapers to be worn by the infant, and mark the weight in grams on the diapers.

EQUIPMENT AND SUPPLIES

- Scale with gram measurement
- Urine toilet collection device, urinal
- Graduated cylinder

PROCEDURE FOR INFANTS *Clean Gloves*

1. When a precise measurement of output for infants is needed, weigh the diaper after the infant has voided or had a stool. Disadvantages to this procedure include the inability to differentiate between urine and stool weights since the two substances may mix in the diaper, and the evaporation of urine that takes place after about 30 minutes.

   RATIONALE: *For each 1 gram increase in weight of the diaper, 1 mL of liquid has been excreted by the infant.*

2. Count the number of wet diapers. The amount of micturition is fairly standard during infancy and early toddlerhood. Four to eight wet diapers per day is usually normal.

3. A urine bag may be used to obtain a fairly accurate measurement. Watch for any leakage. See Chapter 7: Specimen Collection for application of a urine bag.

4. Document the output in the medical record.

PROCEDURE FOR TODDLERS AND OLDER CHILDREN

Once the child is toilet trained, urine is collected in a toilet collection device or urinal. The output is measured as for adults with a graduated cylinder.

See Chapter 7: Specimen Collection for output measurement when a urinary catheter is in place.

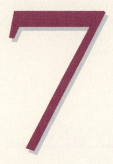

7

Specimen Collection

In the collection of any type of specimen, it is the nurse's responsibility to be sure that the specimen is collected accurately, labeled correctly, and sent to the laboratory using any special techniques or conditions needed such as immediate transport or maintaining on ice. Be sure to review laboratory policy and procedures if you are not familiar with all special criteria.

Blood Samples

There are two methods of obtaining blood samples in children: capillary puncture and venipuncture.

A capillary puncture may be used to obtain a sample for complete blood count, reticulocyte count, platelet count, or blood chemistries such as electrolyte, glucose, or drug levels.

SKILL 7-1 Performing a Capillary Puncture

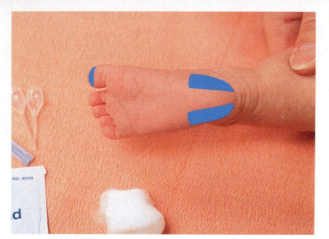

Figure 7-1 *Heel and big toe sites for capillary puncture.*

PREPARATION

1. Explain to the child and parents what will be done and what the child is likely to feel.
2. Applying a hot pack to the collection site before the procedure will increase blood flow and improve results.
3. Have another nurse, an assistant, or the parent ready to restrain the child.
4. Choose the appropriate site. Puncture sites include the plantar surface of the heel (Figure 7-1) (for newborns and children under the age of 1 year), the great toe (for children over 1 year), and the lateral surface of the tip of the third or fourth finger.

EQUIPMENT AND SUPPLIES

- Chlorhexidine-based preparation or other approved skin preparation
- Lancet
- Gauze pads and adhesive bandage
- Appropriate microsize blood collection tubes

CLINICAL TIP

Give newborns concentrated sucrose solutions (12% or 24%) with a pacifier approximately 2 minutes prior to a capillary puncture as a pain relief measure. Sucrose may provide a natural pain relief by activating endogenous opioid systems in the body. The analgesic effect of sucrose lasts approximately 3 to 5 minutes, with a peak action in 2 minutes (Mitchell & Waltman, 2003).

PROCEDURE *Clean Gloves*

1. Apply gloves.
2. *Finger stick.* Hold the child's hand with your nondominant hand (or have an assistant hold it), keeping the finger to be used extended and pointed down.

   Heel stick. Hold the child's foot in your nondominant hand, supporting the dorsum of the foot with your thumb and the ankle with your other fingers.

   Toe stick. Grasp the child's foot across the dorsum with your nondominant hand, supporting the toe with your thumb on the plantar surface.
3. Clean the site with the preferred skin preparation.
4. Using your dominant hand, pierce the skin quickly with the lancet.
5. Wipe the first drop of blood away with the dry gauze.

   RATIONALE: *The first drop may be contaminated by skin contact, and the blood cells may have been traumatized during the stick.*

6. Gently squeeze the site, hold the punctured site downward, and direct the blood into the appropriate tube.

7. When collection is complete, have an assistant hold the gauze on the site until the bleeding has stopped. Apply an adhesive bandage.

8. Document the specimen collected and time sent to the laboratory.

SKILL 7-2 Newborn Screening

Blood screening of the newborn is performed to evaluate blood sugar and to assess for phenylketonuria, hypothyroidism, and other inborn metabolic diseases. A small amount of blood can usually be obtained by heel stick for these tests. The timing of certain tests is important in interpretation of results. Phenylketonuria testing must be done after 24 hours of age for accurate results; metabolic screening is collected before 72 hours of age.

PKU (margin note)

PREPARATION

1. Examine the newborn's record for results of any prior tests.

2. Verify the test and procedures for the specimen to be collected.

3. Explain the procedure to the parents.

4. Wrap a warm washcloth around the foot for a few moments to promote blood flow to the foot and improve blood collection.

EQUIPMENT AND SUPPLIES

- Chlorhexidine-based preparation or other approved skin preparation
- Lancet
- Capillary tube
- Metabolic screening card
- Washcloth rinsed in warm water (optional)

PROCEDURE *Clean Gloves*

1. Don gloves.

2. Clean the site with the preferred skin preparation.

3. Flexing the infant's forefoot up toward the leg (dorsiflexion), use the lancet to puncture the heel, collecting one large drop of blood.

4. The blood may be placed in a capillary tube, onto a metabolic screening card, or onto a glucose reagent strip, depending on the test desired.

5. To place blood on a screening card, completely fill the indicated circles (see Figure 7-2). Insufficient coverage of the circles will result in a need to repeat the test.

6. Allow the paper to air-dry in a horizontal position at room temperature. Alternatively, if the blood is being sent to the laboratory in the capillary tube, seal the open end with Critoseal and transport according to agency policy.

7. Clearly label the blood samples and cards with the newborn's identifying information. Record the day and time, and the child's age in hours.

8. Document the specimen collection and time sent to the laboratory.

> ### COMMUNITY CARE CONSIDERATION
>
> When metabolic screening cards are completed in an office or clinic visit in the first days after birth, the specimen collected must be sent to the laboratory within 24 hours of collection.

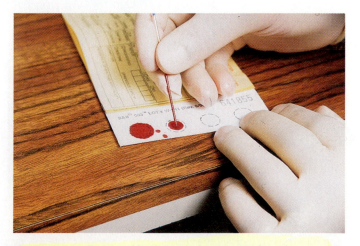

Figure 7-2 *Collecting a blood sample from the newborn for neonatal metabolic screening.*

SKILL 7-3 Blood Glucose Meters

Children with diabetes commonly perform capillary punctures several times daily to measure their blood glucose with a small instrument.

PREPARATION *Clean Gloves*

1. Verify the identity of the child. The procedure is explained to the child and family.

2. The nurse demonstrates the procedure as needed and observes the child or family on return demonstration.

3. The diabetic child is taught over time how to safely perform repeated blood glucose tests and how to maintain materials.

EQUIPMENT AND SUPPLIES

- Reagent strips
- Blood glucose meter
- Alcohol swab
- Lancet

PROCEDURE *Clean Gloves*

1. The child and any assistants wash their hands.
   RATIONALE: *This removes surface contaminants from the child's hands to reduce the chance of infection or false readings (e.g., food residue on fingers).*

2. The assistant dons gloves.

3. Clean the finger to be used with alcohol if desired. This is not necessary for the diabetic patient with repeated tests (Figure 7-3).
   RATIONALE: *With repeated testing, alcohol can cause drying and cracking of the skin. Washing with soap and water removes most surface contaminants.*

4. Milk the finger gently or warm the hand if cold.
   RATIONALE: *This encourages blood circulation to the fingertip so that the sample can be easily obtained.*

5. Quickly puncture the fingertip with the lancet.

6. Apply a drop of blood to the reagent strip.

7. Place the strip into the glucose meter and read the instrument as instructed (Figure 7-4).

8. Document the test results and time collected.

HOME AND COMMUNITY CARE CONSIDERATIONS

Children with diabetes who perform finger sticks for blood glucose analysis should be taught about safe practices for cleaning blood from surfaces by using bleach solution. Safe storage is needed to prevent young children from having access to the lancets. Identify a place in the school where the child can keep glucose-monitoring equipment and perform the procedure in private.

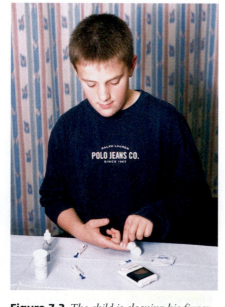

Figure 7-3 *The child is cleaning his finger prior to piercing the skin for blood glucose monitoring.*

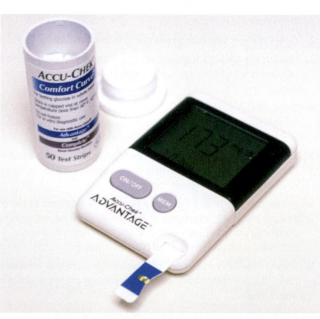

Figure 7-4 *Blood glucose monitors are small and quickly analyze a drop of blood and display the blood glucose in mg/dL.*

SKILL 7-4 Performing a Venipuncture

Venipuncture, or the puncturing of a vein, is used to obtain a sample for complete blood count, blood culture, sedimentation rate, blood type and crossmatch, blood clotting times, drug screen, ammonia level, or fibrinogen level.

PREPARATION

1. Verify the identity of the child. Explain the procedure to the child and parent.
2. Choose the appropriate site. The veins of the antecubital fossa or forearm are usually the best choice because of their accessibility. However, the dorsum of the hand or foot also may be used. (See Figure 9-1B on page 84 for venipuncture site locations.)

EQUIPMENT AND SUPPLIES

- Chlorhexidine-based preparation or other approved skin preparation
- Tourniquet
- 20- to 27-gauge needle with attached syringe (slightly larger than volume of blood needed)
- A butterfly needle may be appropriate for smaller children
- Dry gauze pad and adhesive bandage
- Large-bore (19-gauge) needle
- Appropriate blood collection tubes

PROCEDURE *Clean Gloves*

1. Apply gloves.
2. Place a tourniquet proximal to the desired vein to distend it (Figure 7-5A). If necessary, hold the extremity below heart level, gently rub or tap the vein, or apply a warm compress to promote dilation of the vein.
3. Explain to the child that you are looking for the best vein to use to collect the blood.
4. Locate the vein by inspection (wiping with alcohol will make the vein shine) or by palpation.
5. Once the vein has been located, clean the skin with alcohol or the preferred skin preparation, using an outward circular motion (Figure 7-5B). Let dry. The skin will appear dull.
6. With your nondominant hand, hold the skin taut, gently pulling with your thumb just under the site of the puncture.
7. Puncture the skin with the needle, beveled up at a 15-degree angle and directed toward the vein. When blood appears in the tube, gently pull back on the syringe (Figure 7-5C).
8. Release the tourniquet after all the blood has been collected. Remove the needle at the same angle used for entry, and apply pressure to the site with the dry gauze pad (alcohol will sting).
9. Recognize the child for his or her cooperation.

CLINICAL TIP— VENIPUNCTURE

- Make sure the tourniquet is tight enough to restrict venous but not arterial blood flow.
- Keep the bevel of the needle up.
- Do not draw back too hard or rapidly on the syringe because the vein will collapse.
- If blood fails to enter the syringe, the needle may not be placed correctly in the vein. Advance it slightly.
- If a flash was seen initially but blood no longer appears, the needle may be located incorrectly in the vein. Gently draw back on the needle slightly.

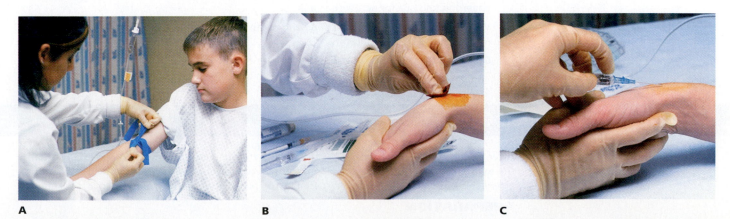

Figure 7-5 *Venipuncture procedure: A, The tourniquet is applied to restrict venous blood flow. B, The area for venipuncture is cleaned by the nurse with the preferred skin preparation and dried with a cotton ball. C, The needle is placed with the bevel up and gently inserted into the identified vein.*

10. Have the assistant or parent maintain direct pressure over the site for a few minutes until the bleeding has stopped, at which point an adhesive bandage can be placed. Meanwhile, discard the needle in a sharps container.

11. Attach the large-bore (19-gauge) needle, and expel blood into the appropriate collection tubes as soon as possible.

12. Document the blood collection and the time sent to the laboratory.

SKILL 7-5 Blood Cultures

Cultures of blood samples may be performed to determine if a child has septicemia. Such samples are commonly drawn two different times a few hours apart to assist in accurate diagnosis of causative microorganisms.

PREPARATION

1. Verify the identity of the child. Explain the procedure to the child and parents.

2. Choose the appropriate site. The veins of the antecubital fossa or forearm are usually the best choice because of their accessibility. However, the dorsum of the hand or foot also may be used. (See Figure 9-1B on page 84 for venipuncture site locations.)

EQUIPMENT AND SUPPLIES

- Chlorhexidine-based preparation or other approved skin preparation
- Tourniquet
- 20- to 27-gauge needle with attached syringe (slightly larger than volume of blood needed)
- Butterfly needle (may be appropriate for smaller children)
- Dry gauze pad and adhesive bandage
- Large-bore (19-gauge) needle
- Appropriate blood collection tubes

PROCEDURE *Sterile Gloves*

1. When infection is suspected, the first blood collection is performed before starting antibiotics.
   RATIONALE: *Antibiotics may alter the results so that a microorganism is not detected.*

2. Apply sterile gloves, and thoroughly cleanse the skin with the approved skin preparation.
   RATIONALE: *Strict sterile technique reduces the chance that skin surface bacteria are found in the laboratory, leading to misdiagnosis.*

3. Use either venipuncture or an arterial line for samples as ordered.

4. Samples at the two different times are usually drawn from different sites.
   RATIONALE: *Results can be compared to determine if microorganisms are present in the blood rather than just from skin contamination during the blood collection.*

5. Each blood collection specimen is split and placed in two different culture tubes—one for anaerobic and one for aerobic bacteria.

6. Verify that specimen labels match patient identification, transport the specimens as recommended by the laboratory.

7. Document the specimen collection and time sent to the laboratory.

SKILL 7-6 Arterial Blood Gases

Arterial blood gas (ABG) analysis is used to monitor the adequacy of ventilation and oxygenation, the oxygen-carrying capacity of the blood, and acid-base levels. ABG samples can be obtained from arterial puncture. At other times the specimen may be collected from an indwelling arterial line.

PREPARATION

1. Explain the procedure to the family and to the child, as developmentally appropriate.

2. Use two methods of identification to verify the identity of the child.

3. Choose the appropriate site. Arterial puncture can be performed on the radial, brachial, and femoral arteries. On newborns, samples are often obtained from the temporal or radial artery. Avoid using the femoral artery because use of this site increases the risk for aseptic necrosis of the femoral head. Arterial samples can also be obtained by deep heel puncture or from an indwelling arterial catheter.

4. Assess the collateral circulation of the extremity to be used for an arterial stick.

EQUIPMENT

- ABG kit or heparinized syringe with 25- to 27-gauge needle and cap
- Anesthetizing agent
- 2″ × 2″ gauze pads
- Adhesive bandage
- Chlorhexidine-based preparation or other approved skin preparation
- Label for specimen
- Ice for specimen transport

PROCEDURE *Clean Gloves*

1. Use developmentally appropriate nonpharmacologic methods to reduce pain and anxiety. If time allows, apply an anesthetizing agent such as EMLA (60 minutes before puncture). Alternatively, at the time of the procedure a vapocoolant spray or intradermal injection of buffered lidocaine can be used to numb the skin.
   RATIONALE: *Arterial punctures are painful. Breath holding and crying can affect the accuracy of blood gas values.*

2. Apply gloves and prepare the site for puncture with the preferred skin preparation.

3. Palpate the artery for puncture, and insert the needle at a 60- to 90-degree angle.

4. Watch for blood backflow into the syringe. Do not pull back on the plunger. Blood should automatically fill the syringe/container due to arterial pressure. Withdraw the required amount of blood into the syringe/container.

5. Withdraw the needle and apply pressure to the site with 2″ × 2″ sterile gauze pad for 5 to 10 minutes.
   RATIONALE: *Pressure must be applied to stop bleeding and prevent hematoma formation.*

6. Place the specimen in an appropriate container and check for air bubbles. Remove air bubbles.
   RATIONALE: *Air bubbles can affect the blood gas values.*

7. Verify that the specimen label matches the child's identification. Label with the child's temperature and percentage of oxygen administered as both affect blood gas values. Place the specimen on ice and send to the lab immediately.
   RATIONALE: *Ice prevents red blood cell metabolism. Blood must be evaluated immediately for accurate results.*

8. Document the procedure including site, results of Allen test (positive if adequate collateral circulation present), amount of blood withdrawn, time sent to the laboratory, and how the child tolerated the procedure.

CLINICAL TIP

The Allen test can be performed to assess collateral circulation of the radial, ulnar, or brachial arteries. Elevate and blanch the extremity distal to the planned puncture site. The two arteries providing blood flow to the limb are then occluded. The extremity is lowered and pressure from one artery is relieved. Color returning to the extremity in less than 5 seconds indicates adequate collateral circulation.

Urine Samples

A urine sample is obtained to assess for infection and to determine levels of blood, protein, glucose, acetone, bilirubin, drugs, hormones, metals, and electrolytes. Urine can also be evaluated for concentration/specific gravity, pH, and crystals or other substances.

A clean-catch or sterile catheter urine specimen is needed to evaluate the presence of microorganisms. The procedure varies according to the developmental level of the child. Infants and young children will have to be catheterized. Older children can often void and provide a midstream voided specimen.

SKILL 7-7 Applying a Urine Collection Bag (Infant)

CLINICAL TIP

When applying the urine bag on girls, begin by placing the bag below the vaginal opening and then allow it to adhere to the labia. For boys, be sure the bag is adhered on the scrotum and the scrotum is not inside the bag's opening. Cutting a hole in the diaper so the end of the bag can pass through makes it easier to visualize when the infant has urinated.

PREPARATION

1. Explain the procedure to the parents.

EQUIPMENT AND SUPPLIES

- Urine collection bag (newborn or pediatric size as needed)
- Soap solution and water or packaged cleansing swabs for cleaning genitalia
- Urine specimen container

PROCEDURE *Clean Gloves*

1. Don gloves.
2. Remove the diaper and clean the skin well, ensuring any skin folds are opened for access to cleaning.
3. Avoid touching the inside of the bag as you handle it.
4. Attach the bag with the adhesive tabs (Figure 7-6): for girls, around the labia; for boys, around the penis.
5. Make sure the seal is tight to prevent leakage.
6. Check the bag frequently for urine.

TO REMOVE A BAG CONTAINING URINE

7. Don gloves.
8. Gently pull the bag away from the skin. Fold the opening over and place the urine bag into the specimen container.
9. Cap the container tightly.
10. Label with name, date, time, and test ordered. Send promptly to the laboratory.
11. Document the specimen collection and time sent.

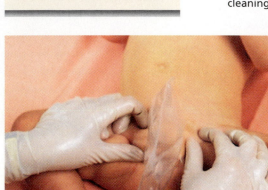
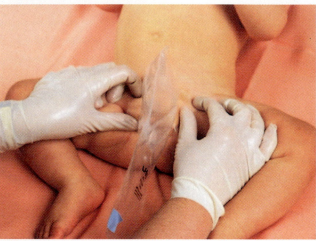

Figure 7-6 *Attaching the urine collection bag.*

SKILL 7-8 Routine Urine Collection (Older Child)

When a sterile sample is not required, the child may void into a container that is placed in the toilet to collect the sample. Don gloves. Pour the urine into the specimen collection cup.

SKILL 7-9 Collecting a Clean-Catch Midstream Urine Specimen (Older Child)

PREPARATION

1. Explain the procedure to the child and parents.

EQUIPMENT AND SUPPLIES

- Towelettes
- Sterile urine specimen container

PROCEDURE *Clean Gloves*

Male

1. Instruct the older child (parent or nurse) to wash hands well, and then clean the head of the penis (after pulling back the foreskin, if not circumcised) three times, each time using a different towelette, moving from the urethral meatus outward. All ridges and skin folds should be cleaned.

2. Have the child begin to urinate a small amount into the toilet and then catch the flowing urine in the sterile container.

3. Cap the container tightly. Always wear gloves in case there are any urine spills on the container.

4. Label with name, date, and time. Send promptly to the laboratory.

5. Document the specimen collection and time sent to the laboratory.

Female

1. Instruct the child (parent or nurse) to wash the hands well. The girl should sit back on the toilet as far as possible with her legs apart. After spreading the labia, wipe each side with a separate towelette using a front-to-back stroke. A third wipe is used to clean the meatus, repeating the front-to-back motion.

2. Have the child urinate a small amount into the toilet and then catch the flow in the sterile container.

3. Cap the container tightly. Wear gloves in case of any urine spills on the container.

4. Label with name, date, and time. Send promptly to the laboratory.

5. Document the specimen collection and time sent to the laboratory.

SKILL 7-10 Collecting a Sterile Urinary Catheter Specimen

PREPARATION

1. Check the physician's orders to determine whether intermittent or indwelling catheterization is planned.

2. Determine the size of the catheter based on the child's size, age, and weight.

3. Confirm the identity of the child and explain the procedure to the child and parent and why it is necessary.

EQUIPMENT AND SUPPLIES

- Urinary catheter—size appropriate for the child's age, and one a size smaller
- Sterile urinary catheterization tray (containing drapes, sterile gloves, antiseptic solution, cotton swabs or balls, forceps, lubricant, and a container for urine)
- Container for soiled cotton balls
- Syringe filled with normal saline
- Tape
- Drainage collection apparatus
- Absorbent pads

> **CLINICAL TIP**
>
> Recommended urinary catheter sizes:
>
> Infant—4–5 French
>
> Toddler and preschooler—6 French
>
> School-age child—6–10 French
>
> Adolescent—8–12 French

PROCEDURE Sterile Gloves

1. Have an assistant hold the child in position for the procedure. If the parents wish to stay with the child, have them stand at the child's head and try to distract the child.

2. Place absorbent pads under the child's perineum.

3. Open the tray, maintaining the sterile field. Open the lubricant and squeeze it onto the sterile field. Pour the antiseptic over the cotton swabs or balls.

4. Put on sterile gloves. Lubricate the tip of the catheter and place the distal end in the specimen container.

Female

1. Clean the perineum. Spread the labia apart with the nondominant hand. Pick up the antiseptic-soaked cotton balls with forceps using the dominant hand. Clean the meatus, using one ball for each wipe, in a front-to-back direction along each side of the labia minora, then along the sides of the urinary meatus, and finally straight down over the urethral opening. Discard each cotton ball away from the sterile field.
   RATIONALE: *Wiping in the direction from the urinary meatus toward the anus avoids contaminating the urinary meatus with fecal bacteria.*

2. Pick up the lubricated catheter tip with your dominant hand, keeping the distal end in the specimen container.

RATIONALE: *The dominant hand remains sterile and should be the one to handle the catheter. Placing the distal end in a specimen container prevents contamination of the sterile field when urine flows.*

3. Gently insert the catheter tip into the meatus (approximately 5 to 8 cm [2 to 3 in] in the child) until there is a free flow of urine, and then 2.5 cm (1 in) further. If resistance is felt, do not force the catheter. Gently try to rotate the catheter between your fingers and try to advance. If unsuccessful in advancing the catheter, try again with another sterile catheter, preferably one size smaller.

   RATIONALE: *A catheter should not be used a second time to prevent potential infection in the child.*

4. When the catheter is in place, collect the urine specimen and drain the bladder while holding the distal end of the catheter with the nondominant hand. Remove the tube.

5. Cap the container tightly. Always wear gloves in case there are any urine spills on the container.

6. Label with name, date, and time. Send promptly to the laboratory.

7. Document the specimen collection and time sent to the laboratory.

Male

1. Clean the perineum. With the nondominant hand, hold the penis behind the glans and spread the meatus with your thumb and forefinger. Retract the foreskin if the child is uncircumcised.

2. Use the dominant hand to pick up the forceps and antiseptic-soaked cotton balls. Clean the tissue surrounding the meatus using one cotton ball for each wipe in an outward circular motion. Discard each cotton ball away from the sterile field.

3. Pick up the lubricated catheter tip with the dominant hand, and place the distal end in a specimen container. Lift the penis, exerting slight traction until it is perpendicular to the body. Insert the catheter steadily into the meatus until urine begins to flow, and then about 2.5 cm (1 in) further (up to a total of 10 to 12 cm [5 to 6 in] maximum) (Figure 7-7).

   RATIONALE: *The catheter is inserted an extra inch into the bladder to ensure proper placement for drainage when an indwelling catheter is planned.*

4. If resistance to the catheter is felt, have the child blow out to relax the perineal muscles, or rotate the catheter between your fingers and gently advance. Do not force the catheter. Another catheter, one size smaller, may be used if relaxation efforts are not successful.

5. Once the catheter is in place, lower the penis and collect the urine specimen while holding the distal end of the catheter with the nondominant hand. Remove the tube.

6. Cap the container tightly. Always wear gloves in case there are any urine spills on the container.

7. Label with name, date, and time. Send promptly to the laboratory.

8. Document the specimen collection and time sent to the laboratory.

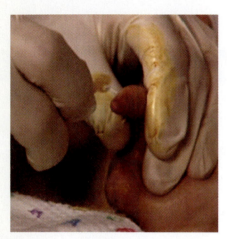

Figure 7-7 *Performing urinary catheterization in a male infant.*

SKILL 7-11 Collecting an Indwelling Catheter Urine Specimen

PREPARATION

1. Explain the procedure to the child and parent if present.

EQUIPMENT AND SUPPLIES

- Clamp
- Alcohol swab
- Syringe with needle
- Sterile specimen container

PROCEDURE *Clean Gloves*

1. Locate the self-sealing port on the urinary catheter tubing. The site is distal to the balloon that is inserted to keep the catheter in place.

   RATIONALE: *Self-sealing rubber catheters have a port that can be accessed with a syringe. This technique cannot be performed on plastic or silicone catheters. The port is distal to the balloon to avoid puncturing and dislodging the catheter.*

2. Wash hands and apply gloves.

3. If there is no urine in the catheter, apply the clamp and wait for several minutes.

4. Clean the port with an alcohol swab.
   RATIONALE: *This minimizes the chance of transferring contaminants from the catheter surface into the urinary tract.*

5. Insert the syringe hub or needle on the syringe into the port at an angle. Release the clamp if it was applied.

6. Withdraw urine and transfer to a sterile specimen container. Discard the syringe in a sharps container.

7. Label with name, date, time, and test ordered. Send promptly to the laboratory.

8. Document the specimen collection and time sent to the laboratory.

SKILL 7-12 Collecting a 24-Hour Urine Specimen

PREPARATION

1. Confirm the identification of the patient and explain the collection procedure to the family and child as developmentally appropriate. Assist the family to choose a 24-hour time frame that is best for them and their child.

2. Document medications the client is taking and identify which could affect the test results.

EQUIPMENT AND SUPPLIES

- Labeled plastic container for urine collection (to be stored in refrigerator or on ice)
- Urine collection container for toilet or urinal
- Funnel
- Urine bags for infants
- Skin sealant such as Skin-Prep if not medically contraindicated (for infants wearing urine bags)

PROCEDURE *Clean Gloves*

1. Assist the child to urinate at the beginning of the 24-hour collection period, and note the time. *Discard this urine.*

2. Record the start time on a labeled collection container.

3. For the next 24 hours, collect all urine in the collection container. Girls may void into the collection container in the toilet and use the funnel to pour urine into the plastic container. Boys may void directly into the collection container or other urine collection container. Urine should not be mixed with stool or toilet paper as these may affect test results. The collection container must be kept refrigerated or on ice. Care must be taken to obtain all the urine.
   RATIONALE: *The test evaluates protein levels per a 24-hour period to measure kidney function. Accuracy of the test depends on obtaining all urine within a 24-hour time frame.*

4. In anticipation of the end of the urine collection after 24 hours, let the child know when the final urine sample will be needed. At the end of the 24-hour period, ask the child to void and record the time the specimen was obtained. This is the stop time for specimen collection.

5. Verify that the specimen label matches the child's identification and test to be performed. Record the stop time on the urine collection container.

6. Send urine in the collection container promptly to the laboratory.

7. Document the procedure and time sent to the laboratory.

Stool Culture

Stool cultures are used to detect the presence of bacteria and other organisms in the intestinal tract. A sample for culture can be obtained from stool collected in a cup, from a diaper, or from a swab that has been gently inserted into the child's rectum. A test for parasites requires larger size samples and is usually submitted in a stool specimen cuplike container.

SKILL 7-13 Obtaining a Stool Specimen

PREPARATION

1. Gather supplies.
2. Explain the procedure to the child and parents.

EQUIPMENT AND SUPPLIES

Two culturette swabs or a stool specimen container and two tongue blades

PROCEDURE *Clean Gloves*

1. Don gloves.
2. Open one culturette swab, holding it in your dominant hand while keeping the cover in your nondominant hand. If the swab is attached to the cover, hold the culturette tube in the nondominant hand and the swab and cover in the dominant hand.
3. Dip the swab into the stool. Replace the cover. Squeeze the bottom of the closed culturette to release the culture medium. Some laboratories will want the entire specimen sent in a sterile specimen collection cup.
4. Repeat with the second culturette.
5. Label with name, date, time, and test ordered. Promptly send to the laboratory.

FOR PARASITIC AND OTHER SPECIMENS

1. Don gloves.
2. Obtain the specimen from a diaper or toilet collection device by using tongue blades.
3. Place the specimen in a stool container.
4. Label the container with name, date, time, and test requested. Send to the laboratory immediately for parasite examination.

Wound Culture

A culturette swab is used to obtain samples for microscopic examination from a wound or body site such as the eyes, ears, nose, throat, rectum, or vagina.

SKILL 7-14 Obtaining a Sample for Wound Culture

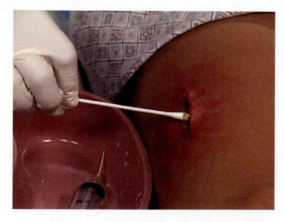

Figure 7-8 *Collecting a wound culture with a culturette swab.*

PREPARATION

1. Gather supplies.
2. Explain the procedure to the child and parents.

EQUIPMENT AND SUPPLIES

One culturette swab

PROCEDURE *Sterile Gloves*

1. Don sterile gloves.
2. Open the culturette, holding it in the dominant hand while keeping the cover in the nondominant hand. If the swab is attached to the cover, hold the culturette tube in the nondominant hand and the swab and cover in the dominant hand.
3. Gently swab the infected area (Figure 7-8).
4. Place the swab into the culturette tube. Squeeze the tube to release the culture medium.
5. Label with name, date, time, site of culture, and test requested. Promptly send to the laboratory.
6. Document the specimen collected, site collected from, and time sent to the laboratory.

Throat Culture

A culturette swab is used to obtain a sample from the throat for microscopic examination.

SKILL 7-15 Obtaining a Sample for a Throat Culture

PREPARATION

1. Verify the identity of the child. Explain the procedure to the child and parents.
2. Gather supplies.

EQUIPMENT AND SUPPLIES

- Two culturette swabs
- Penlight
- Tongue blade

PROCEDURE *Clean Gloves and Mask*

1. Don gloves and mask.
2. Open the culturette, holding it in the dominant hand while keeping the cover in the nondominant hand. If the swab is attached to the cover, hold the culturette tube in the nondominant hand and the swab and cover in the dominant hand.
3. Use the penlight as needed to provide adequate views of the throat.
4. Gently swab the back of the throat along each tonsillar area with a separate culturette.
5. Place the swab into the culturette tube. Squeeze the tube to release the culture medium.
6. Label the specimen with name, date, and time. Promptly send to the laboratory.
7. Document the specimen collected and time obtained.

> **CLINICAL TIP**
>
> Throat cultures must be properly performed for accurate diagnosis. A sterile cotton-tip applicator is swabbed across the tonsils, posterior edge of the soft palate, and uvula. Cooperative children can be asked to put their hands under their buttocks, open their mouth, and laugh or pant like a dog. The throat is quickly swabbed. Uncooperative and young children are placed on their back with their hands next to their head and held by a parent or an assistant. The tongue is gently depressed with a tongue blade, and the throat is swabbed.

Respiratory Secretions

Secretions are obtained to detect bacteria that cause respiratory infections. Different techniques are used for infants and older children. The infant will need suctioning. The older child can cooperate and cough into the provided container.

SKILL 7-16 Collecting Respiratory Secretions from an Infant

PREPARATION

1. Explain the procedure to the parents.
2. Gather supplies.

EQUIPMENT AND SUPPLIES

- Sterile suction catheter
- Sterile normal saline
- Suction trap
- Personal protective equipment (mask, gown, eye protection)

PROCEDURE *Sterile Gloves, Droplet Precautions*

1. According to the manufacturer's guidelines, attach the suction trap to low wall suction (60 mm Hg).
2. Apply gown, mask, eye protection, and sterile gloves.
3. Suction the child's nose (refer to the description of suctioning in Chapter 11), using a small amount of sterile normal saline to clear the tubing.

> **CLINICAL TIP**
>
> A common respiratory infection in young children is caused by respiratory syncytial virus (RSV). In young children the course of disease can be severe. Cultures may be taken to identify the disease in infants so that proper treatment can be instituted.

4. Close the trap.

   NOTE: *This will provide a specimen from the nasopharyngeal area. If a tracheal specimen is needed, the deep suctioning technique described in Chapter 11 should be consulted.*

5. Label the specimen with name, date, time, and test ordered. Promptly send to the laboratory.

SKILL 7-17 Collecting Respiratory Secretions from a Child

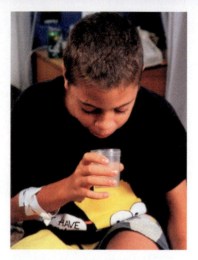

Figure 7-9 *Child supplying a sputum specimen.*

PREPARATION

1. Verify the identity of the child. Explain the procedure to the child and parents.
2. Gather supplies.

EQUIPMENT AND SUPPLIES

- Sterile specimen container

PROCEDURE *Clean Gloves (Mask may be needed)*

1. Don gloves and mask.
2. Encourage the child to take several deep breaths and then cough sputum up and spit it directly into the cup (Figure 7-9).
3. Have the child close the cup.
4. Label the specimen with the name, date, time, and test ordered. Promptly send to the laboratory.
5. Document the specimen collected and time sent.

Bone Marrow Aspiration

The bone marrow is the tissue that manufactures the blood cells. The marrow should contain hematopoietic cells (blood forming), fat cells, and connective tissues. A bone marrow aspiration (and/or biopsy) is performed as a diagnostic procedure for the diagnosis and staging of hematologic disorders or cancers or to harvest bone marrow for transplant. Examination of the aspirate or biopsy specimen may also reveal infections. For a bone marrow aspiration, a thin needle is used to extract a small amount of liquid bone marrow. For a bone marrow biopsy, a small cylinder of bone and marrow is removed with a needle. Common pediatric sites for bone marrow aspiration are the posterior iliac crest, the anterior tibia, and the sternum.

A physician generally performs the aspiration, and the nurse assists with the procedure by positioning the child, preparing the child and family, and monitoring vital signs and response to the procedure prior to, during, and following the aspiration.

SKILL 7-18 Assisting with Bone Marrow Aspiration

PREPARATION

1. Verify the identity of the child. Explain the procedure to the parents and child.
2. Assess for any special medical problems or conditions that may complicate the procedure.
3. Gather proper specimen sample supplies, equipment, and pain and sedation medications (lidocaine hydrochloride, EMLA cream).
4. Apply a local anesthetic agent well in advance of the procedure.

EQUIPMENT

- Gown, sterile gloves, mask worn by physician performing aspiration
- Sterile cotton balls or gauze
- Sterile forceps
- Sterile drape
- Stack of sterile 4×4 and 2×2 gauze pads
- Chlorhexidine-based, povidone-iodine, or other preferred skin preparation
- Sterile gloves, nonsterile gloves
- Spinal needles
- Sheet or towel roll for patient positioning
- #11 blade
- Bone marrow aspiration needles (16 gauge, 1¾ or 2 inch) or Jamshidi bone marrow biopsy needles (11 to 13 gauge)
- Sterile 10-mL and 20-mL syringes for sample procurement
- Specimen tubes, containers, and microscope slides with proper preservatives and fixatives, sealed container for biopsy
- Sodium heparin, injection, 1000 USP units/mL
- Adhesive bandage or elastoplast tape for pressure dressing
- Pulse oximetry for monitoring the sedated child
- Oxygen, resuscitator bag, and emergency equipment and medications immediately available

> ### CLINICAL TIP
> Bone marrow aspiration is a painful procedure. Effective sedation and pain management is important to reduce the child's anxiety. Positive coping with this event will facilitate management of future painful procedures.

PROCEDURE

1. Assist with assembling the supplies and preparing the room. Verify that consent has been signed.
2. Assist with the preparation, positioning, and immobilization of the patient to provide optimal access to the aspiration site. Take baseline vital signs. Administer sedation and pain medication if prescribed.
3. Follow the guidelines for patient monitoring before and throughout the procedure and until the child is fully responsive following the procedure. Monitor for signs of distress or excess pain.
   RATIONALE: *The child is often sedated for the procedure and needs to have vital signs carefully monitored.*
4. If the child is awake during the procedure, provide diversion or coping support.
5. After the site of the bone marrow aspiration is selected, the skin is cleansed and prepared, and the local anesthetic is applied or injected (the skin and periosteum are infiltrated with lidocaine 1%).
6. The skin is punctured at the insertion site with the #11 blade, and the bone marrow aspiration needle is inserted into the bone (Figure 7-10A).
7. The stylette is removed and syringes are attached to withdraw marrow (Figure 7-10B).
8. Samples are placed in the appropriate containers with labels, and needed preservatives are added.
9. After cleansing the site, apply a bandage.
10. Document the test performed, site used, vital signs and pulse oximetry readings, how the child tolerated the procedure, signs and symptoms of bleeding, and the time the specimen was sent to the lab.

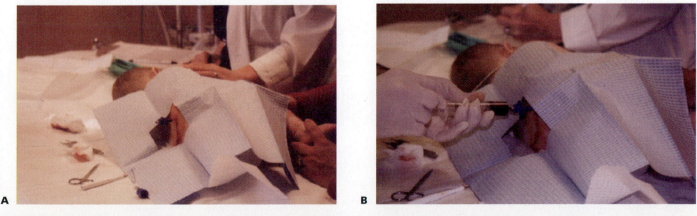

A **B**

Figure 7-10 *Bone marrow aspiration: A, Insertion of the bone marrow needle into the posterior iliac crest. B, Aspiration of bone marrow.*
Photos donated by the Family of Barrett Thomas Harris.

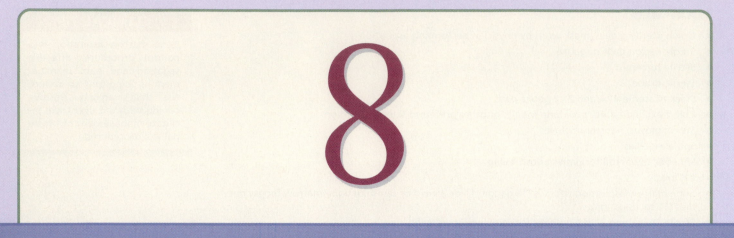

Administration of Medication and Irrigations

Administration of Medication

Administering medications to children presents a number of challenges: deciding which drug forms to use, determining dosages, choosing methods and sites, and taking into account implications based on the child's development. See Table 8-1 for considerations needed when administering medications to children by various routes.

TABLE 8-1	Variations in Medication Administration to Children	
Route	**Developmental Considerations**	**Techniques**
Oral	Children under 5 years cannot generally swallow pills and capsules.	■ Medications are usually given in liquid form (e.g., elixir, syrup, or suspension). ■ Use a tuberculin syringe to measure amounts less than 1 mL to increase accuracy. ■ Sometimes tablets are crushed or capsules are opened and mixed with one spoon of food. Check with pharmacy to be sure this does not inactivate the drug. Never crush enteric-coated or timed-release medicine. ■ When choosing a vehicle for crushed tablets, use only one spoonful of applesauce, pudding, jelly, or similar food so that it is easier to ensure that the entire dose will be taken.
	Children may not want to take medicine.	■ Position young children upright to avoid choking and aspiration. ■ Give liquid medicines slowly by oral syringe (for infants) aimed at the inside of the cheek or by medicine cup (for toddler and preschooler) for drinking. ■ Communicate with the child that you expect that the medicine will be taken. Let children choose the type of fluid to drink after but do not ask if they will take their medicine now.
Rectal	Colon is small in size.	■ Lubricate the tip of the suppository before placement. ■ Place the suppository at the rectal opening and advance past the sphincter. ■ For children under 3 years, the nurse's gloved fifth finger is used for insertion. After this age the index finger can usually be used.
Ophthalmic and otic	Young children may be fearful of medicines placed in the eyes or ears.	■ Adequate restraint is needed to avoid injury. ■ The nurse's hand can be stabilized by resting the wrist on the child's head. ■ Explanations and therapeutic play can be used with children old enough to explain the process of administration. ■ Have medication at room temperature.
Topical	Skin of infants is thin and fragile.	■ Only prescribed doses and medicines appropriate for young children should be used on the skin. ■ Covering the area or keeping the child's hands occupied may be necessary to ensure adequate contact of medication with the skin.
Intramuscular	Anatomy and physiology of children differs from that of adults.	■ The gluteus maximus muscle (dorsal gluteal site) must not be used until the child has been walking for at least 1 year. ■ The vastus lateralis site is preferred for young children. ■ Amounts to be administered should be limited to no more than 1–2 mL for ventrogluteal site depending on muscle size. ■ The deltoid muscle is rarely used in young children except for the small amounts injected in some vaccines.
Intravenous	Veins are small and fragile.	■ Careful maintenance of sites is needed. ■ Common infusion sites include hands and feet, although scalp veins are sometimes used in infants.
	Fluid balance is critical.	■ Infusion pumps require frequent monitoring. ■ Syringe pumps are often used to administer medications when minimal fluid is to be given. ■ Central lines are commonly used for long-term intravenous medication therapy.

"6"

TABLE 8-2	"Five Rights" of Medication Administration

1. Right medication
   - Compare the name and concentration of the drug on the medication sheet with the name and concentration of the drug on the label of the drug container three times. Check the container's expiration date.
   - Know the action of the drug.
   - Identify the potential side effects of the drug.
   - Use the pharmacy, hospital, or other drug formulary as a reference for medications with which you are unfamiliar.
2. Right patient
   - Verify the name, medical record number, and date of birth on the medication sheet with these items on the child's identification band. When in a setting with no name band (e.g., clinic), verify the child's name and date of birth with the child and parent by asking them to state the name and date of birth.
3. Right time
   - When prescribed to be administered at a specific time, a medication should be given within 20–30 minutes of that time.
   - For prn medications, check the last time the dose was given as well as the total 24-hour dose the child has received to verify that the child can receive another dose at this time.
4. Right route of administration
   - Always use the prescribed route for administration of a medication. If a change is needed (such as a change from oral medication when a child is vomiting), check with the prescriber to get an order for a change in route.
   - If a verbal order must be taken, read back the order to the prescriber to verify accuracy.
5. Right dose
   - Match the dose and concentration with the order.
   - Calculate the prescribed dose based on the child's weight in kilograms.
   - If in doubt about what constitutes an appropriate dose, compare with the pharmacy, hospital, or other drug formulary guidelines for recommended dose.
   - Question any order for which the dose is outside of recommended amounts.

6. Documentation

Although the drug and the dosage are determined by the prescriber, it is imperative that the nurse observe the "~~five~~ rights" of medication administration before any medication is given (Table 8-2). *6*

Preparation

- Explain all procedures or treatments to the child and parents, based on the child's developmental stage, cultural considerations, limited English proficiency (LEP), and the level of understanding of both parties.
- Confirm the medication prescription and the identity of the child.
- Answer all questions before giving the medication.
- Identify any known drug allergies and prior reactions to medication.
- Match the drug available to the medication prescribed and check the expiration date.
- Observe the medication for intactness (tablet/capsule), clarity, and color change; discard and seek new medication as needed.

Documentation

- Once a medication is given, record the name of the drug, the route, the date and time, and, if appropriate, the site.
- Record the response to the medication, including desired effects and undesired side effects. Design observations to coincide with the drug's onset and peak action times.
  RATIONALE: *A record of response is especially important with medications for pain control and those for treatment of an acute problem such as respiratory difficulty.*

Calculation

It is the nurse's responsibility to calculate the dosage of the medication prescribed to determine if the dosage is within the normal range for the child's height and weight.

Dosages can be calculated using the child's weight (written as mg/kg) or total body surface area. This is determined by plotting the child's height and weight on a nomogram (see Appendix C). Draw a line connecting the two columns, and note the results at the point where the drawn lines cross the center column. The dosage is ordered as mg/m^2.

Example 1

The physician prescribes morphine (available as 10 mg/mL) for a 3-year-old child who weighs 15 kg. The recommended dose for children is 0.1 mg/kg. What dose is appropriate for the child's weight? How much volume should be drawn?

Answer

Recommended dose × Weight = Dose for patient

0.1 mg/kg × 15 kg = 1.5 mg

Dose desired/Dose on hand × Quantity in mL = Volume to be administered

1.5 mg/10 mg × 1 mL = 0.15 mL to be administered

Example 2

The physician prescribes phenobarbital (65 mg/mL) for a 5-year-old child who weighs 20 kg. The recommended loading dose for the child is 10 to 20 mg/kg. The physician prescribes 250 mg to be infused over 30 minutes. Is this dose appropriate for the child's weight? How much volume should be drawn? How do you set the infusion pump?

Answer

Recommended dose × Weight = Desired dose

10 mg/kg × 20 kg = 200 mg

20 mg/kg × 20 kg = 400 mg

Dose of 250 mg is within recommended range.

Dose desired/Dose on hand × Quantity in mL = Volume to be administered

250 mg/65 mg × 1 mL = 3.85 mL

Pump Setup

Using recommendations from the manufacturer, the nurse determines that the volume of fluid needed to infuse the medication is 50 mL.

50 mL/30 min × 60 min/1 hr = mL/hr = 100 mL/hr

Rate = 100 mL/hr

Oral Medication

Children younger than 5 years of age usually have difficulty swallowing tablets and capsules. For this reason, most medications for pediatric use are also available in the form of elixirs, syrups, or suspensions. If a medication is only available in tablet or capsule form, it may need to be crushed before being administered. Be sure not to crush medications with enteric coating. Remember to wear clean gloves if your hands might come in contact with the child's saliva.

SKILL 8-1 Administering an Oral Medication

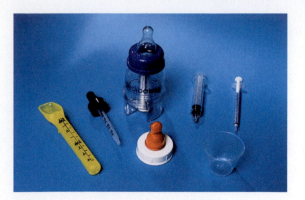

Figure 8-1 *Oral medications can be administered with various types of equipment, depending on the child's age.*

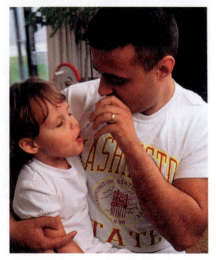

Figure 8-2 *This father needs to administer a medication to his daughter at home. He has been instructed how to hold her and administer the dose safely and effectively.*

PREPARATION

1. Verify concentration, dose, and route as described previously.
2. Measure the medication accurately to ensure that the dose is correct.
3. If the oral medication is liquid (especially if less than 5 mL), it should be measured in a syringe or calibrated small medicine cup or dropper (Figure 8-1). A specially designed medication bottle may also be used.
4. If a tablet or pill needs to be crushed, place it in a mortar or between two paper medicine cups and crush it with a pestle. Once the tablet or pill has been pulverized, mix the powdered medication with a small amount of flavored substance such as juice, applesauce, or jelly to disguise any unpleasant flavor.
5. Verify identification of the child to receive the medication.
6. Explain the procedure to the parent. State the name of the drug to be given.

EQUIPMENT AND SUPPLIES

- Medicine cup, oral syringe, or other device for administering medication
- Pestle and medicine cups
- Medication
- Mixing medium as needed, such as applesauce

PROCEDURE *Clean Gloves*

Infant

1. A syringe or dropper provides the best control.
2. Apply gloves if needed.
3. Place small amounts of liquid along the side of the infant's mouth. Wait for the infant to swallow before giving more.
   RATIONALE: *This helps to prevent aspiration and maximizes the chance that the infant will get all the medicine rather than spitting some out.*
   Alternative method: Have the infant suck the liquid through a nipple.
4. Document administration of the medication and both expected and side effects.

Toddler or Young Child

1. Place the child firmly on your lap or the parent's lap in a sitting or modified supine position (Figure 8-2).
2. Apply gloves if needed.
3. Administer the medication slowly with a syringe or small medicine cup.
4. Document administration of the medication and both desired and side effects.

Intramuscular Injection

The site of the intramuscular injection (Figure 8-3) depends on the age of the child, the amount of muscle mass, and the density and volume of medication to be administered. Young infants may not tolerate volumes greater than 0.5 mL in a single site, whereas older infants or small children may be able to tolerate 1 mL per site. As the child grows, greater volumes can be administered.

Note: The larger the volume of medication, the larger the muscle to be used. Avoid areas that involve major blood vessels or nerves.

The preferred site for the infant is the vastus lateralis muscle (Figure 8-4), which lies along the midanterior lateral aspect of the thigh. After the child has been walking for 1 year, the dorsogluteal site can be used. However, since the muscles in this area are poorly developed and since the sciatic nerve is difficult to avoid, it is not the ideal choice for a child less than 5 years old.

VLC
Very little children

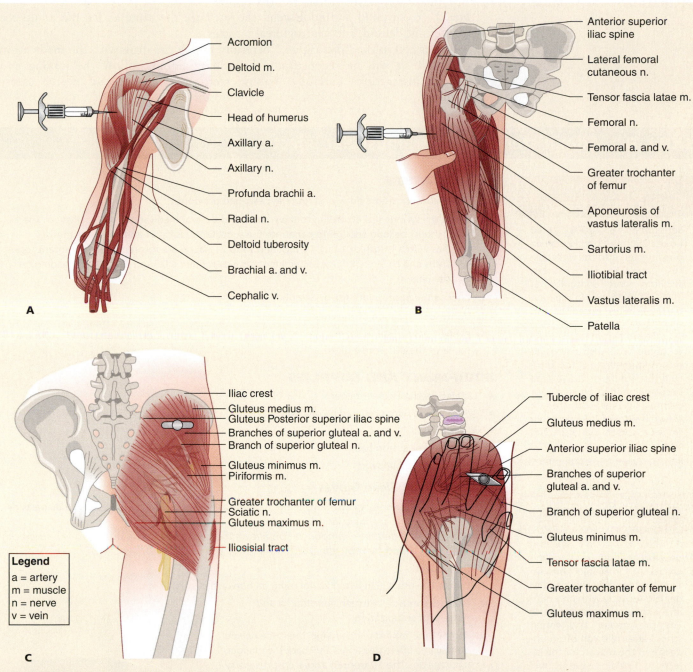

A

Acromion
Deltoid m.
Clavicle
Head of humerus
Axillary a.
Axillary n.
Profunda brachii a.
Radial n.
Deltoid tuberosity
Brachial a. and v.
Cephalic v.

B

Anterior superior iliac spine
Lateral femoral cutaneous n.
Tensor fascia latae m.
Femoral n.
Femoral a. and v.
Greater trochanter of femur
Aponeurosis of vastus lateralis m.
Sartorius m.
Iliotibial tract
Vastus lateralis m.
Patella

C

Iliac crest
Gluteus medius m.
Gluteus Posterior superior iliac spine
Branches of superior gluteal a. and v.
Branch of superior gluteal n.
Gluteus minimus m.
Piriformis m.
Greater trochanter of femur
Sciatic n.
Gluteus maximus m.
Iliosisial tract

Legend
a = artery
m = muscle
n = nerve
v = vein

D

Tubercle of iliac crest
Gluteus medius m.
Anterior superior iliac spine
Branches of superior gluteal a. and v.
Branch of superior gluteal n.
Gluteus minimus m.
Tensor fascia latae m.
Greater trochanter of femur
Gluteus maximus m.

Figure 8-3 *Intramuscular injection sites. A, Deltoid. B, Vastus lateralis. C, Dorsogluteal. D, Ventrogluteal.*
Redrawn and modified from Bindler, R., & Howry, L. (2005). *Pediatric drug guide with nursing implications* (pp. 41–44).
Upper Saddle River, NJ: Prentice Hall Health.

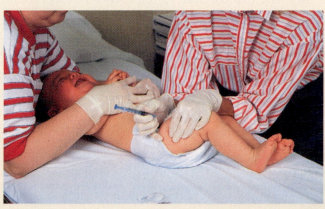

Figure 8-4 *In infants, the vastus lateralis muscle is preferred for intramuscular injections.*

For the older child and adolescent, the sites are the same as for the adult: the vastus lateralis, deltoid, and ventrogluteal muscles.

As described in the "five rights," carefully match the drug with the medication prescribed. If it will be reconstituted by adding liquid, follow the mixing and calculation instructions carefully. Follow sterile procedures and needle safety precautions.

SKILL 8-2 Administering an Intramuscular Injection

SAMPLE DOCUMENTATION FROM A CLINIC SETTING

September 6, 2005, 1400 hours: 250 mg (1 mL) ceftriaxone injected into the right vastus lateralis. No redness, swelling noted. September 6, 2005, 1420 hours: No reaction to medication noted at this time. Vital signs stable (see flowsheet). Patient discharged to home with instructions to return immediately for difficulty breathing or if the area becomes red, swollen, or painful. Further instructed to return if signs of infection continue or worsen. Signature and title of nurse.

GROWTH AND DEVELOPMENT CONSIDERATIONS

Consider the child's age and developmental level when preparing for IM injections. Infants and toddlers will need to be held securely with only minimal explanations understood. The preschooler and young school-age child can often understand the reason for the injection. Explain what it will feel like, such as "I am going to clean your arm now with alcohol. This feels cold but does not hurt." And then, "You will feel the stick now and it's OK to tell me if it hurts." Children also can benefit from distractions that help them to manage the injection. "When I give the shot, let's count to ten together. OK, it's in—one, two, three. . . ." And finally, praise children for some part of their behavior. "I know you were scared but you held very still so we could do it fast."

PREPARATION

1. Verify concentration, dose, and route as described previously.
2. Select the syringe size according to the volume and dose of medication to be delivered. The needle must be long enough to penetrate the subcutaneous tissue and enter the muscle. Needles with a length of 1 to 1 1/2 inch and 25 to 21 gauge are recommended for infants over 4 months and children. Infants under 4 months may require a 0.5-inch needle, depending on muscle mass.
3. Choose the appropriate site as described previously.
4. Verify identification of the child.
5. Explain the procedure to the parent and to the child if old enough to understand. State the name of the drug to be given.

EQUIPMENT AND SUPPLIES

- Labeled medication container
- Syringe filled with prepared medication
- Alcohol swab
- Gauze pad or cotton ball
- Small adhesive bandage

PROCEDURE *Clean Gloves*

1. Have another nurse, an assistant, or the parent position and hold the necessary body parts of the child during the injection (Figure 8-5).
   RATIONALE: *Adequate immobilization allows the procedure to be done safely and quickly and thereby minimizes trauma for the child.*
2. Don gloves.
3. Locate the site. Clean with alcohol using an outward circular motion.
4. Grasp the muscle between your thumb and fingers for stabilization.
5. Remove the cap from the syringe. Insert the needle quickly at a 90-degree angle. Pull back the plunger.
   RATIONALE: *The 90-degree angle ensures entry into the muscle when the needle length is adequate. Pulling back of the plunger helps to rule out placement in a blood vessel.*
6. If no blood is aspirated, inject the medication, withdraw the needle, massage the area with a gauze pad or cotton ball (alcohol will sting), and return the child to a position of comfort. Apply a small adhesive bandage if there is a drop of blood visible.
7. Do not recap the needle. Discard it in a puncture-resistant container according to standard precaution recommendations.
8. Document the medication administration, site, and reactions of the child.

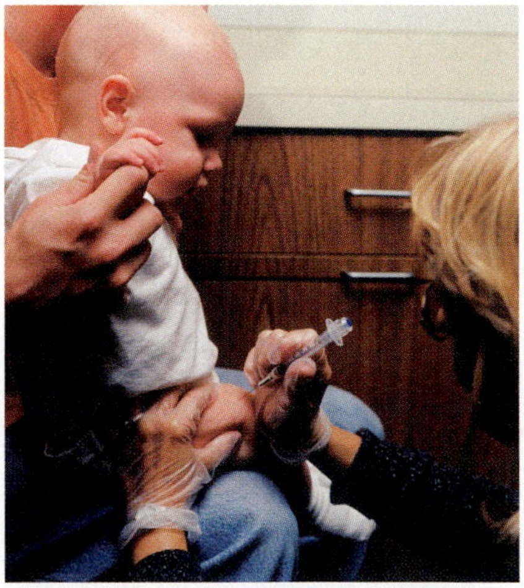

Figure 8-5 *The infant's legs and arms are controlled by the father and nurse so an injection can safely be administered.*

Subcutaneous Injection

The site of the subcutaneous injection depends on the age of the child. Usually the dorsum of the upper arm or the anterior thigh is used in newborns, infants, and toddlers.

SKILL 8-3 Administering a Subcutaneous Injection

PREPARATION

1. Verify concentration, dose, and route as described previously.
2. Select the syringe size based on the volume or dose of medication to be delivered. The needle must be just long enough to penetrate the subcutaneous tissue, which lies below the skin and fat surface and above the muscle. Needles with a length of 3/8 to 5/8 inch (26 to 25 gauge) are recommended for infants and children.
3. Choose the appropriate site as described above.
4. Verify identification of the child.
5. Explain the procedure to the parent and to the child if old enough to understand. State the name of the drug to be given.

EQUIPMENT AND SUPPLIES

- Labeled medication container
- Syringe filled with medication
- Alcohol swab
- Gauze pad or cotton ball
- Small adhesive bandage

PROCEDURE *Clean Gloves*

1. Have another nurse, an assistant, or the parent position and hold the necessary body parts of the child while the injection is being given.
2. Don gloves.
3. Locate the site. Clean with alcohol using an outward circular motion.
4. Pinch the skin between your thumb and index finger.
5. Remove the cap from the syringe. Insert the needle quickly at about a 45-degree angle. Release the skin and pull back the plunger.
   RATIONALE: *A 45-degree angle is used to inject into the subcutaneous tissue rather than the underlying muscle.*
6. If no blood is aspirated, inject the medication, withdraw the needle at the angle at which it was inserted, massage the area with a gauze pad or cotton ball (alcohol will sting), and return the child to a position of comfort. Apply an adhesive bandage if there is a drop of blood present.
7. Do not recap the needle. Discard it in a puncture-resistant container according to standard precaution recommendations.
8. Document the medication administration, site, and reactions of the child.

Intravenous Medication

The principles of intravenous (IV) medication administration in children are the same as those in adults. Special considerations when administering IV medication are discussed in this section. Accessing lines when a medication lock is in place or a central line is used is discussed in Chapter 9.

Many drugs have specific dilution recommendations. Some medications are compatible with only specific fluids such as normal saline. Other medications must be given very slowly. Still other drugs can be administered quickly. Know your agency or pharmacy standards for IV push or bolus administration (less than 10 minutes) versus intermittent medication administration. Be sure you know which medications are incompatible with one another and with types of IV fluids.

Special Considerations

It is recommended that IV medications for infants and children be put in a volume control chamber such as a Soluset or Metriset with the diluent and placed on an electronic pump for accurate administration. Alternatively, a syringe pump may be used, especially when fluid intake is closely regulated. Set the pump for the volume to be infused and the rate of infusion. Check the pump frequently to detect malfunction. Flush the line after the infusion to ensure that all medication has been administered, since some medication will remain in the distal tubing. Consult agency policy for an acceptable flush solution.

SKILL 8-4 Administering an Intravenous Medication

PREPARATION

1. Review the medication, the administration recommendations, and the child's former responses and drug allergies.
2. Assess the IV line for patency.
3. If you are administering narcotics or benzodiazepines, have antagonists and ventilation equipment at the bedside.
   RATIONALE: *The effect of most IV medications is almost immediate.*
4. Prepare the drug according to the order and manufacturer guidelines. Reconstitution or withdrawal of solution from a vial or ampule may be needed.
5. Identify the child and explain the procedure to the child and family. State the name of the drug to be given.

EQUIPMENT AND SUPPLIES

- Labeled medication container
- Syringe and needle or needleless system
- Prepared medication
- Dilution solutions
- Alcohol swabs

PROCEDURE *Clean or Sterile Gloves*

1. Assess IV line for patency and side effects. If the child has a medication lock in place, flush the line with 2 to 5 mL normal saline to check for patency or insert the IV line and allow to run for several minutes. Check the site again. See Chapter 9 for further details.
2. Identify the port on the IV line to be used for push medications or for insertion of a syringe pump. Generally a port proximal to the child is used, especially for intermittent infusion.
   RATIONALE: *A proximal port ensures that the medication will be delivered at the time administered. When an IV line is running slowly, it may take some time for the medication to travel from a distal port into the child.*
3. Identify the medication port on the volume control chamber for intermittent infusion.
4. Don gloves.
5. Clean the port and surrounding tubing with an alcohol swab and allow to air dry.
   RATIONALE: *Cleansing minimizes the chance of instilling harmful organisms into the IV line.*
6. Insert the needle or needleless syringe for IV push medication. While watching the time, slowly insert the medication in the ordered time frame. Observe the child carefully during administration. Stop the infusion if the child suddenly becomes lethargic or hyperactive, demonstrates changes in respirations or color, or has other rapid changes in behavior or appearance.
   RATIONALE: *Since IV push medications travel quickly into the vein, side effects can appear rapidly. Close observation is needed to prevent and respond quickly to undesired effects.*

SAFETY PRECAUTIONS

It is recommended that needleless systems be used whenever available to decrease the chance of needlestick injuries to patients and healthcare providers.

SAFETY PRECAUTIONS

It is important that tubing for IV administration and tubing and syringes for IV medication administration have no air. Prime tubing properly so air does not get injected into the child's vein. This could be harmful to the child. Verify carefully what lumen to use when the child has a line with multiple lumens.

7. When using a syringe pump, insert the primed tubing into a port close to the child. Set the infusion time as prescribed for the medication.

8. When using intermittent medication administration, insert the medication in the proper dilution in the volume control chamber. Regulate the pump to administer the medication in the desired time.

   RATIONALE: *Medications should be administered in recommended time frames to ensure safety and effectiveness. Most antibiotics are administered over 30 to 60 minutes.*

9. Check on the child's condition several times during administration.

   RATIONALE: *Monitoring ensures that the child with side effects is identified and that the IV infusion is patent and running on time.*

10. At the end of administration, flush the tubing with normal saline or by running IV fluid.

    RATIONALE: *Flushing ensures that the entire amount of medication is infused and not left in the tubing. Flushing also removes medication from the line so that it will not mix with other drugs administered.*

11. Document administration and effects observed. Assess the IV line and document findings.

Ophthalmic Medication

The first ophthalmic medication is given as prophylaxis for sexually transmitted infection in the newborn. The procedure is described in Skill 8-5. Older children receive ophthalmic medication for treatment of infections and other eye conditions, and the technique for administration is described in Skill 8-6. Children usually fear having anything placed in their eyes, and special care is often needed to reduce the child's anxiety and promote cooperation during instillation of ophthalmic medications. An explanation of the procedure may help gain the child's cooperation. To prevent the transfer of pathogens to the eye, the medication and its dispensing port must be kept sterile.

SKILL 8-5 Administering Neonatal Ophthalmic Ointment

Gonorrhea, *Chlamydia,* and *Staphylococcus aureus* can colonize within the birth canal without symptoms in the mother. The infective agents can be transferred to the newborn during birth and lead to eye infection which is called ophthalmia neonatorum. Application of erythromycin ophthalmic ointment can prevent this infection and protect eyesight. It is easy to administer and causes few side effects. For this reason it is applied soon after birth following drying of the newborn, attending to temperature, assessing initial adaptation, and ensuring adequate oxygenation. Eye prophylaxis is required by law in the United States and Canada; it can be declined in writing by parents in Canada.

PREPARATION

1. Gather necessary supplies.
2. Verify the identity of the newborn.
3. Teach parents about the medication and the reason for administration.

EQUIPMENT AND SUPPLIES

- Clean cotton pads
- Sterile gloves
- Erythromycin ophthalmic ointment

PROCEDURE *Sterile Gloves*

1. Perform hand hygiene. Swaddle the infant and place in a supine position.

   RATIONALE: *Swaddling the infant will help to keep hands from interfering with medication administration.*

2. Don gloves. Using a cotton pad, wipe excess fluid and vernix from one eye, working from the inner to outer canthus.

3. Repeat with the opposite eye using a clean cotton pad.

4. Remove gloves and perform hand hygiene. Open the medication.

5. Don gloves.

6. Stand at the infant's head.

7. Using thumb and fingers of the nondominant hand, retract both the upper and lower eyelids so that the eye can be visualized (Figure 8-6A).

8. Apply a 1- to 2-cm (half inch) line of ointment into the lower conjunctival sac, working from the inner to outer canthus. Be careful not to touch the tube to the eye or mucous membrane.

9. Repeat on the opposite eye, maintaining sterile application technique.

10. Refrain from wiping the eyes after administration.

11. Document administration in the medical record.

SKILL 8-6 Administering an Ophthalmic Medication

PREPARATION

1. Gather supplies.

2. Verify the medication order with the available medication.

3. Identify the child and explain the procedure to the child and family. State the name of the drug to be given.

EQUIPMENT AND SUPPLIES

- Medication
- Sterile gloves

PROCEDURE *Sterile Gloves*

1. Have another nurse, an assistant, or the parent hold the child's upper body in a supine position with the child's head extended.

2. Don gloves.

3. Use your nondominant hand to pull the child's lower lid down while your other hand rests on the child's head (Figure 8-6B).

4. Instill the drops or ointment into the conjunctival sac that has formed.
   Alternative method: Pull the lower lid out far enough to form a reservoir in which the medication can be instilled.

5. After the medication has been instilled, close the child's eyelids to prevent leakage.

HOME CARE CONSIDERATIONS

Instilling Eye Medications
It can be challenging to safely instill eye medication into young children. Give parents the following suggestions:

- Perform hand hygiene.
- Be sure the medicine is warmed to room temperature.
- Remove any drainage from the eye with a clean or sterile moist, warm cloth or gauze.
- Wash your hands again.
- Have the child lie on the back with eyes closed.
- Gently pull the lower lid down to form a small pocket.
- Apply a thin string (for ointment) or drops of the medicine.
- Allow the eyelid to return to the normal position.
- Have the child keep the eye closed for several seconds.
- Help prevent spread of the infection by keeping the child's hands clean.
- Enhance comfort by keeping the head elevated to decrease swelling and avoiding exposure to bright light.

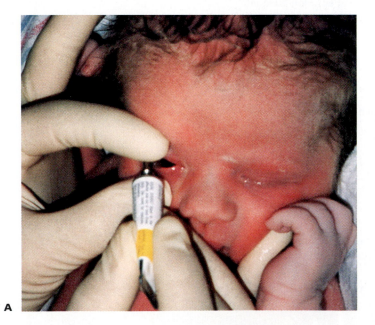

A

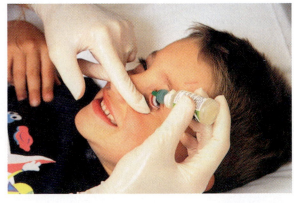

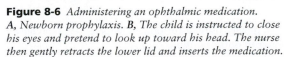
B

Figure 8-6 *Administering an ophthalmic medication.*
A, Newborn prophylaxis. B, The child is instructed to close his eyes and pretend to look up toward his head. The nurse then gently retracts the lower lid and inserts the medication.

6. Have the child lie quietly for a minimum of 30 seconds. Discourage the child from squeezing the eyes shut.

7. Dry the inner canthus of the eye.

8. Keep the child's head in the midline position to prevent the medication from contaminating the other eye.

9. Document the medication administration and the child's response.

10. When the child requires ophthalmic medication at home, instruct parents in proper technique.

Contact Lens Care

When children are hospitalized or receiving healthcare, providers should ask if contact lenses are used. Follow the prescriber's and family's directions for care of contact lenses. Encourage the child and family to care for lenses whenever possible. General guidelines include the following:

- Keep the lenses in the eyes for the recommended time only.
- Store each lens in the right or left containers as labeled.
- Wash hands carefully before contact with the child's eyes or lenses.
- Use a cleaning solution on the lens after its removal.
- Rinse the lens with the recommended rinsing solution.
- Keep the lenses in the case with the disinfecting storage solution.
- Note on the chart that the child wears lenses.

Eye Irrigation

Irrigation of the eye is performed to flush out a foreign body or a chemical irritant (Figure 8-7). Children often close the injured eye tightly, so getting them to relax for this procedure is important. Care must be taken not to touch the cornea, which could cause further eye injury. Careful aseptic technique is needed to prevent infection.

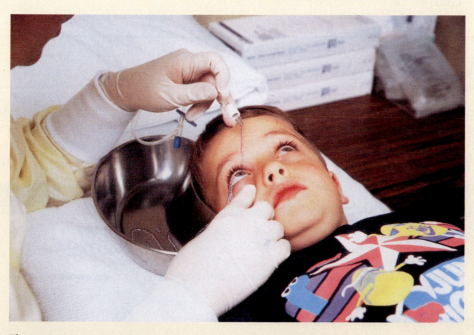

Figure 8-7 *Eye irrigation.*

SKILL 8-7 Performing an Eye Irrigation

PREPARATION

1. Check the prescriber's orders for the type of fluid and the volume to be used (most often sterile normal saline).

2. Identify the child and explain the procedure to the child and family.

3. The child will need to be held in position for this procedure. An assistant can hold the child supine, keeping the child's head turned slightly so that the eye to be irrigated is lower than the other eye, and being sure that the child has free exchange of air.
   RATIONALE: *This method is used to avoid cross-contamination of the eye not being irrigated.*

4. Attach the IV tubing to the bag of room-temperature normal saline. Purge the line, but keep the tip covered.

EQUIPMENT AND SUPPLIES

- Absorbent pads
- Irrigation solution and tubing
- Basin

PROCEDURE *Sterile Gloves*

1. Place absorbent pads under the child's head, neck, and shoulders, using towels for extra absorption. Place an emesis basin under the lower eye to catch drainage.

2. Don gloves.

3. Using the thumb and forefinger of your dominant hand, gently separate the child's lids.

4. Remove the cover from the IV tubing. Open the clamp midway, pointing the stream of fluid into the lower conjunctival sac from the inner to the outer canthus. Periodically turn off the stream of solution and have the child close the eye.
   RATIONALE: *This allows the solution to also move into the upper conjunctival area.*

5. When the irrigation has been completed, dry the child's eye gently with gauze or a cotton ball from the inner to the outer canthus.

6. Assess the return for color, odor, and character. Observe the irrigation solution and eye for a foreign body.

7. Document the treatment and the child's response.

Otic Medication

Otic medications, which are available in liquid form, are placed in the external ear canal using a dropper. They include antibiotics and pain medications. Otic drops are sometimes applied to soften cerumen, enabling it to be cleansed from the canal. The ear canal is not treated with sterile technique unless the tympanic membrane is ruptured and draining.

SKILL 8-8 Administering an Otic Medication

PREPARATION

1. Gather supplies.

2. Identify the child and explain the procedure to the child and family. State the name of the drug to be given.

EQUIPMENT AND SUPPLIES

- Medication
- Cotton ball

PROCEDURE *Clean Gloves*

1. Have another nurse, an assistant, or the parent hold the child in a supine position with the head turned as appropriate for administration, and ensuring free air exchange (Figure 8-8).
2. Don gloves.
3. For the child less than 3 years of age: Gently pull the pinna straight back and downward to straighten the ear canal. For the older child: Pull the pinna back and upward.
4. When the pinna is in the proper position, instill the drops into the ear.
5. Keep the child in the same position for a few minutes. Gently rub the area just anterior to the ear to facilitate drainage of the medication into the ear canal. If desired, a cotton ball may be loosely placed in the ear for about 5 minutes to promote retention of the medication.
6. Document the treatment and the child's response.

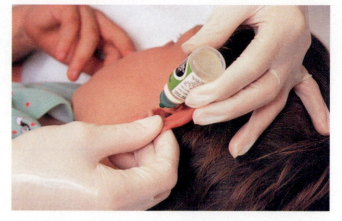

Figure 8-8 *Administering an otic medication.*

Ear Irrigation

Irrigation of the ear is performed to remove cerumen or a foreign body. Frequently the child has symptoms of otitis media but the canal cannot be visualized. Always ask the parent if there has been any drainage from the ear and examine the ear with an otoscope. See your textbook for a description of proper use of the otoscope and normal ear landmarks. If there is drainage, contact the prescriber before irrigating the ear. Be sure to check the auditory canal with the otoscope after each 1 minute of irrigation to observe the effects of treatment.

SKILL 8-9 Performing an Ear Irrigation

PREPARATION

1. Check the prescriber's orders for the type of fluid to be used and the ear to be irrigated.
2. Identify the child and explain the procedure to the child and family.

EQUIPMENT AND SUPPLIES

- Ordered solution, warmed to room temperature
- Irrigating syringe (bulb or Asepto) with tubing, ear irrigation machine, or Waterpik according to agency policy
- Clean gloves
- Absorbent pads
- Basin

PROCEDURE *Clean Gloves*

1. Examine the ear with an otoscope.
   RATIONALE: *The tympanic membrane should be intact before the irrigation is performed.*
2. Place the child in a supine position with the affected ear facing upward. Don gloves. For the child less than 3 years of age, gently pull the pinna straight back and slightly downward. For the older child, pull the pinna back and upward.
   RATIONALE: *These maneuvers straighten the ear canal.*
3. Protect the child's clothing. Place a waterproof pad on the bed under the head. Place an emesis basin under the ear to be irrigated (Figure 8-9).
4. Draw 20 mL of warm ordered solution into a syringe with the tubing attached.
5. Gently flush the solution into the ear canal, catching the draining fluid with the emesis basin. Gently turn the head toward the affected ear to facilitate drainage of the fluid.

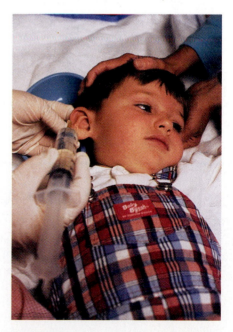

Figure 8-9 *Ear irrigation. Note that the affected ear is facing upward for the instillation of fluid; the head will be rotated toward the bed so that the fluid can drain out after the irrigation is completed.*

6. Alternatively, use an ear irrigating machine or a Waterpik at the lowest setting to flush the ear.

7. Repeat according to the prescriber's orders.

8. Dry the child's ear, cheek, and neck.

9. Reexamine the ear with an otoscope and record changes noted. Document the treatment and the child's response.

Nasal Medication

Medications instilled into the nares drain into the back of the mouth and throat, and may cause sensations of difficulty in breathing, tickling, or bad taste. After instillation of the drops, the child should be observed for choking or vomiting. Saline nose drops are sometimes given to young infants who have respiratory disorders to clear the nasal passages.

SKILL 8-10 Administering a Nasal Medication

EQUIPMENT AND SUPPLIES
- Medication
- Clean gloves

PROCEDURE

1. Verify the identity of the child and explain the procedure to the child and family. State the name of the drug to be given.

2. Place the child in a supine position with the head hyperextended over the parent's lap or over the edge of the examination table or bed.

3. Perform hand hygiene and don gloves.

4. Instill the drops into the nostrils.

5. Keep the child in the same position for at least 5 minutes to allow the medication to contact the nasal mucosa.

6. Document the treatment and the child's response.

Aerosol Therapy

Aerosol therapy is used when a medication needs to be deposited directly into the airway. Bronchodilators, steroids, and antibiotics can be administered to children in aerosol form. Several methods are used to provide aerosol therapy, including mist tents with medications added to a reservoir, intermittent positive pressure breathing machines, or nebulizers. The most common aerosol therapy for children is the metered dose inhaler (MDI) commonly used in treatment of asthma. See your textbook for a description of this treatment for asthma. Since nebulizers are a type of aerosol treatment commonly used in both the hospital and home, and are commonly administered by nurses, their use is also described here.

SKILL 8-11 Administering Nebulizer Aerosol Therapy

PREPARATION

1. The dose of the medication is based on the child's weight. The medication is placed in the cup of the aerosol kit; 2 to 3 mL of normal saline can be added as a diluent if ordered.
2. Perform a baseline assessment, including heart and respiratory rates, peak flow, breath sounds, and respiratory effort.
3. Verify the identity of the child and review or explain the procedure to the parent and child.

EQUIPMENT AND SUPPLIES

- Reservoir
- Mouthpiece, mask, or blow-by tubing (depending on child's age)
- Portable nebulizing machine or tubing to hook to oxygen supply

PROCEDURE

1. Place the mask on the child, have the child put the mouthpiece in his or her mouth (Figure 8-10), or provide an assistant or the parent the tubing for blow-by.
2. Attach the oxygen tubing to the oxygen flow meter at 6 to 7 L/min or use a portable compressor.
3. Have the child take deep breaths during the treatment.
4. The aerosol administration should last about 10 minutes. Reassess the child's condition after the therapy.
5. Document the treatment and the child's response.

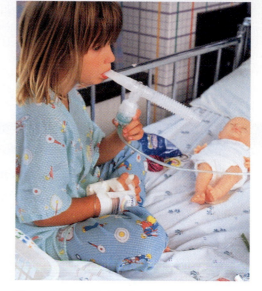

Figure 8-10 *This child has been taught to use a nebulizer for treatment of her asthma in the hospital. After explanation and demonstration by the nurse, she now independently and effectively completes the treatment.*

Metered Dose Inhaler (MDI)

MDIs are small canister devices with a mouthpiece used to treat asthma in the home setting. They may be used on a regular basis or during times of respiratory distress.

SKILL 8-12 Using a Metered Dose Inhaler (MDI)

EQUIPMENT AND SUPPLIES

Inhaler with medication

PROCEDURE

1. Verify the identity of the child and review or explain the procedure to the parent and child.
2. Insert the canister into the mouthpiece.
3. Have the child take a deep breath of room air, inhaling and exhaling completely.
4. Ask the child to close the lips tightly over the MDI mouthpiece and then to inhale deeply and slowly through the mouth.
5. Depress the canister one time while the child is inhaling; one dose of medication will be inhaled.
6. Have the child hold his or her breath for about 5 to 10 seconds to enable medication to reach the lungs.
7. MDIs may have reservoirs, spacers, or extenders attached for those children having difficulty holding their breath long enough or closing their mouths securely over the mouthpiece.
8. Document the procedure and the child's response.

> **CLINICAL TIP**
>
> Some medications are provided in a dry powder inhaler (DPI). These inhalers are activated when the child takes a breath. No spacer is used. Children 5 years and older may be able to use a DPI.

Topical Medication

Topical medications are available in gels, pastes, creams, lotions, and liquid form. They are placed directly on the skin and affected area to relieve or prevent a patient's symptoms. Topical medications are easily absorbed through the skin of young children due to their thin skin and increased vascularity. Topical administration provides treatment to the affected area without wide systemic exposure to the medication, often avoiding broad side effects.

SKILL 8-13 Administering Topical Medication

PREPARATION

1. Verify the medical prescription.
2. Check the expiration date on the medication.
3. Identify the child and explain the procedure to the parent and child.
4. Assess the patient and family's developmental, cognitive, and cultural needs for education since topical medications are often administered at home.
5. Review if there has been any problem with this or similar medications in the past.

EQUIPMENT AND SUPPLIES
(MAY BE CLEAN OR STERILE PROCEDURE)

- Medication
- Skin cleansing supplies: basin, warm water and soap or cleanser, cleansing cloth or gauze
- Absorbent pad, if needed
- Appropriate applicator—sterile tongue blade or cotton swabs or the nurse's gloved hand may be indicated
- Container, if small amount of medication to be applied needs to be removed from larger, primary container
- Dressing (gauze, Tegaderm, tape, etc.) as needed

PROCEDURE *Clean or Sterile Gloves*

1. Position the child to permit access to the affected area. Assistance may be needed to hold the child during the application.
2. Assess the skin area or wound.
3. Using the basin, water, and cloth, gently cleanse the skin if intact. Use sterile gauze for open areas to remove debris from the affected area as ordered.
4. Dry the skin well using gentle padding with gauze.
5. Apply the proper amount of medication and spread over the skin as prescribed. Avoid an excess amount to prevent toxicity.
6. Apply a dressing over the site if indicated. Young children may need a dressing to cover and protect the site.
7. For transdermal patches, apply to a clean, dry, flat surface. Do not cut patches to adjust the dose. Rotate sites to ensure proper absorption.
8. Document the procedure and the child's response.

Rectal Medication

Rectal administration is sometimes used when the oral route is contraindicated. Although absorption is less reliable than with oral preparations, many medications such as acetaminophen, aspirin, antiemetics, analgesics, and sedatives come in suppository form.

SKILL 8-14 Administering a Rectal Medication

PREPARATION

1. If the suppository is to be halved, cut it lengthwise.

2. Verify the identity of the child and explain the procedure to the parent and child. State the name of the drug to be administered.

EQUIPMENT AND SUPPLIES

- Water-soluble lubricant
- Suppository
- Clean gloves

PROCEDURE *Clean Gloves*

1. Have another nurse, an assistant, or the parent hold the child in a side-lying or (if small enough) a prone position on the parent's lap.

2. Don gloves.

3. Slightly lubricate the tapered tip of the suppository. Using either the index finger (in children over 3 years of age) or the little finger (in infants and toddlers), gently insert the suppository into the child's rectum, just beyond the internal sphincter.

   RATIONALE: *Lubrication provides for easy insertion and minimal trauma to the mucous membranes. The child's rectum is small in size. Insertion past the sphincter allows the medication to stay in place for absorption.*

4. Hold the buttocks together for 5 to 10 minutes, until the urge to expel the medication has passed.

5. Document the procedure and the child's response.

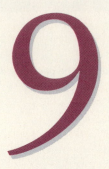

Intravenous Access

Peripheral Vascular Access

In both infants and children, veins of the extremities are used for venous access. Scalp veins may also be used in infants.

Over-the-needle catheters (19 to 27 gauge) are preferred for infants and children. The size of the catheter is determined by the size of the child and the size of the vein. For example, a 24-gauge catheter is used for a newborn; a 20- to 22-gauge catheter is used for an older infant, toddler, or school-age child. A butterfly needle (23 gauge) may be used in certain situations, such as when accessing a scalp vein in an infant or during an emergency for peripheral access in a toddler. Use of a butterfly needle should be considered a temporary measure, with continued effort made to achieve more stable and secure venous access.

Choice of Site

Scalp

Scalp veins are used when other access cannot be obtained (Figure 9-1A). Protect the site by covering it with a plastic medication cup secured with tape.

Extremities

Veins of the antecubital fossa or forearm are usually the best sites for venous access because they are highly visible; however, the dorsum of the hand and foot also may be used (Figure 9-1B).

Special Considerations

- Use foot veins as a last resort for sites in children who are walking.
- Avoid using the child's dominant hand or the hand used by an infant for finger sucking or blanket holding.
- If two sites are needed, do not use both antecubital veins because the child will be rendered unable to flex either arm.
- Use padded armboards as splints to decrease mobility of the extremity.
- Use gauze under tape or tape over tape to decrease skin contact with adhesive tape.

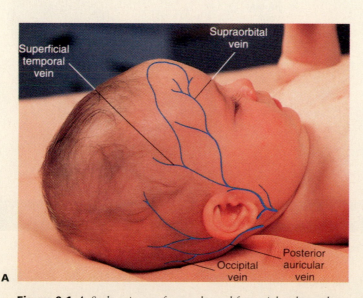

Figure 9-1 *A, Scalp veins are frequently used for peripheral vascular access in infants.*

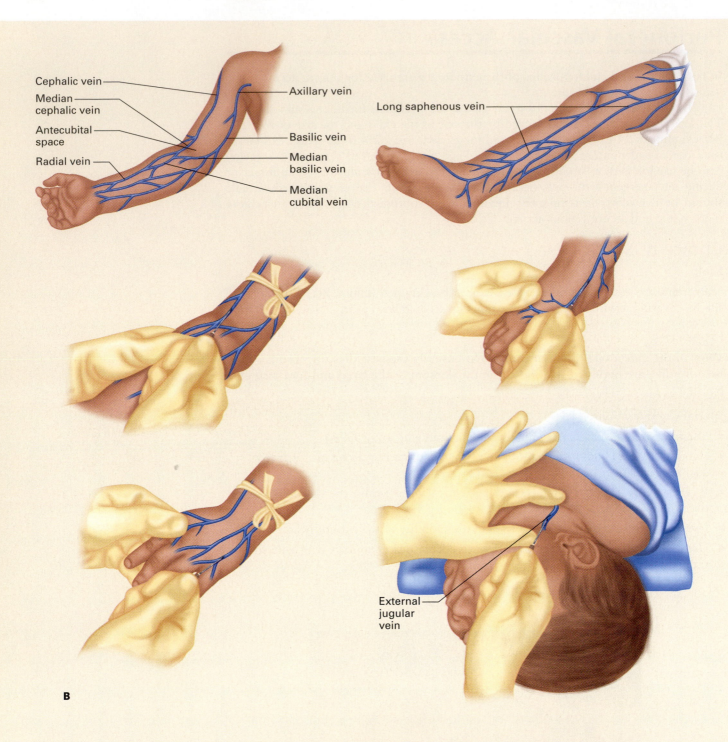

Figure 9-1—Continued B, *Peripheral veins that may be accessed for intravenous administration of drugs and fluids are those of the arms, hands, legs, and feet plus the external jugular vein.*

SKILL 9-1 Accessing a Peripheral Vein

PREPARATION

1. Verify the order for intravenous start and solution, and gather supplies.

2. Place and maintain the child in a supine position with the help of an assistant, or have an older child sit in a chair with the arm on a padded table. Have the person assisting you

lean over the child to control the child's body and extend the extremity to be used. An alternative to human immobilization is to use a papoose board (see Chapter 4).

3. Identify the child and explain the procedure to the child and parent.

EQUIPMENT AND SUPPLIES

- Tourniquet
- Chlorhexidine, alcohol, or povidone-iodine per agency policy
- Different sized armboards
- Over-the needle IV catheter or butterfly needle (select appropriate gauge for size of vein)
- T connector that has been flushed and attached to a normal saline-filled syringe
- IV tubing and bag with solution
- Tape, gauze, transparent dressing

PROCEDURE *Clean Gloves*

1. If a scalp vein is to be used, place a rubber band around the infant's head to serve as a tourniquet to distend the veins. If the extremities are to be used, place the tourniquet proximal to the desired vein to distend it. If necessary, hold the extremity below heart level, gently rub or tap the vein, or apply a warm compress to promote dilation of the vein.

2. Locate the vein by inspection (wiping with alcohol will make the vein shine) or by palpation.

3. If you are using an extremity, apply an armboard or footboard. Relocate the vein.

4. If using the antecubital fossa: Slightly hyperextend the child's elbow and pronate the arm. Secure the arm to the armboard by applying tape above the elbow and at the wrist.

5. If using the dorsum of the hand: Place the child's hand on the armboard, palmar side down, with the fingers wrapped around the distal edge (Figure 9-2). Apply tape over the fingers, then around the thumb separately. Next apply tape at the wrist. A gauze roll may be placed under the wrist to increase flexion.
   RATIONALE: *Positioning to avoid injury is an important nursing role.*

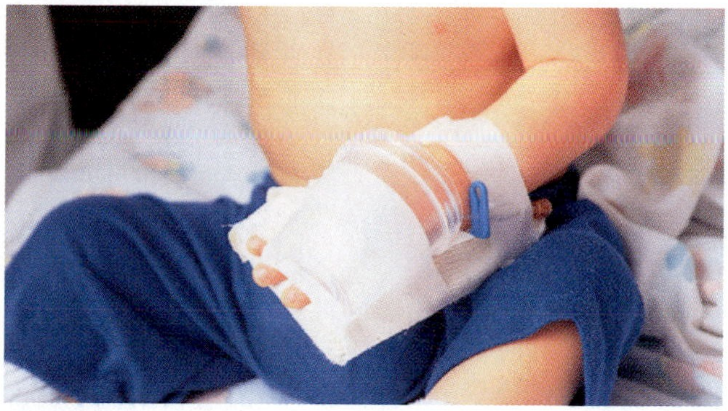

6. If using the foot: Apply the footboard to the child's foot, which is dorsiflexed. Apply tape across the toes, instep, and ankle. Use gauze as needed under the lateral malleolus.

Figure 9-2 *This intravenous site on a hand has been placed on an armboard, securely wrapped, and covered with a plastic protector to prevent the child from disrupting the line.*

7. Clean the skin with chlorhexidine, alcohol, or povidone-iodine per agency policy using an outward circular motion. Let each area dry before continuing. Apply the tourniquet. Hold the skin taut, gently pulling with your thumb just distal to the site of the puncture.

8. Puncture the skin with the catheter, with the bevel side up, positioned at a 15-degree angle and aimed at the vein in the direction of the blood flow. When blood appears, gently slide the catheter into the vein. Release the tourniquet. Remove the stylette.

9. Attach the normal saline-filled T connector and attempt to flush the catheter. If it flushes easily, apply a transparent dressing over the site, and wrap with gauze and stockinette to maintain the site. Alternatively, tape the catheter in place, using a V pattern around the catheter itself, and then secure the catheter with gauze and tape (taking care not to cover the area proximal to the site completely).
   RATIONALE: *Wrapping techniques promote intactness of the line and allow for visualization of the site for signs of infiltration or phlebitis.*

10. Write the date, time, catheter size, and your initials on a piece of tape and place it on the dressing.
    RATIONALE: *Agencies set policies about how long an IV line can be kept in place. Accurate documentation and labeling ensure changes on schedule to avoid infections.*

11. The T connector can be hooked up to a heparin lock or used immediately for fluid or medication infusion.

12. Document the procedure and the child's response, as well as the present assessment of the intravenous site.

See Chapter 7 for further explanation of intravenous access to obtain a blood sample.

Medication Lock

The medication lock is a small device placed on the IV catheter and taped in place. It maintains the IV site for future use when not hooked up to a running IV infusion. Some agencies use normal saline, whereas others use heparin solution to maintain patency of medication locks (this is more commonly done with older children than with infants). Know and follow your agency policy.

SKILL 9-2 Attaching a Medication Lock Cap to an IV Infusion

PREPARATION

1. Verify the order.
2. Verify the identity of the child and explain the procedure to the child and parents.
3. Record intake of intravenous fluid for documentation.

EQUIPMENT AND SUPPLIES

- Syringe filled with 1 mL of prepackaged heparin flush solution (10 units/mL)
- Syringe with 2 mL of sterile normal saline
- Luer-Lok male adapter

PROCEDURE *Clean Gloves*

1. Don gloves.
2. Prime the adapter (fill it, being sure to prevent air pockets) with the heparin flush solution. Maintain sterility of the adapter tip that will be inserted into the intravenous line.
3. Save the rest of the heparin flush solution to use when the lock is inserted into the IV tubing.
4. Be sure the IV line is securely taped in place (Figure 9-3A). Check the patency of the IV tubing by flushing with 2 mL of sterile normal saline. Be sure there is no redness, swelling, pallor, coolness, or pain at the IV site.
5. Clamp the T connector on the IV line to prevent outflow of blood.
6. Remove the IV tubing from the line and quickly place a primed catheter cap on the T connector.
7. Open the clamp. Insert the heparin flush solution or saline and slowly flush the adapter.
8. Remove the syringe and clamp the medication lock.
9. Secure the medication lock with tape and cover with an elastic bandage (Figure 9-3B).
10. Flush the line every 8 hours with heparin flush or saline solution or as determined by agency policy.
11. Document the procedure and the child's response.

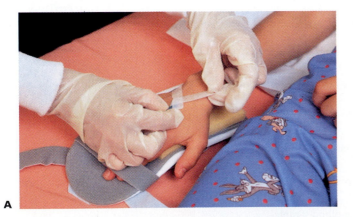
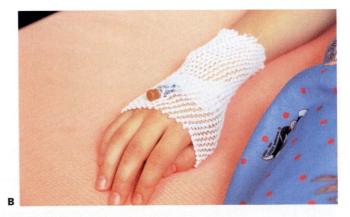

A   **B**

Figure 9-3 *A, Taping the IV line for placement of a medication lock. B, Medication lock in place.*

SKILL 9-3 Infusing Medication: Medication Lock in Place

PREPARATION

1. Check the order.
2. Calculate and verify the medication dosage and concentration.
3. Verify the identity of the child and explain the procedure to the child and parent.

EQUIPMENT AND SUPPLIES

- Alcohol swabs
- 19- to 27-gauge needle or needleless system
- Two syringes filled with 2 mL of normal saline with 19- to 27-gauge needles or needleless system
- Medication ordered
- Syringe with 1 mL of heparin flush solution (10 units/mL) or sterile normal saline

PROCEDURE *Clean Gloves*

1. Prepare the medication to be administered and don gloves.
2. Clean the catheter cap with alcohol. Unclamp the medication lock.
3. Check the patency of the IV tubing by flushing it with normal saline. Check the catheter tip site for swelling.
4. If the IV line is patent and operating, apply the new syringe or needleless system on the distal end of the IV tubing through the cap after cleaning its surface.
   RATIONALE: *Recessed needles or needleless systems are recommended whenever available to promote safety.*
5. Secure the IV tubing and connection area in place with tape.
6. Administer the infusion of medication according to the prescription.
7. Be sure to follow the infusion with 10 to 20 mL of IV fluid so no medication remains in the tubing.
8. After completion of the infusion, discard used equipment into a puncture-proof container according to standard precaution recommendations.
9. If the IV tubing is to be used again, cover it with a clean needle system to ensure sterility.
10. Clean the catheter cap with alcohol.
11. Flush first with 2 mL of normal saline and follow with the heparin flush solution if heparin is to be used (as in the preceding procedure). Clamp the medication lock and secure it in place.
12. Document the procedure and the child's response.

> **RESEARCH CONSIDERATIONS**
>
> Several nursing studies have been performed to measure the effectiveness of heparin versus saline flushes for intravenous lines in children. Different findings and conclusions have failed to give clear guidance to nurses and agencies about the best method. Therefore, agencies may set different policies about this procedure. Evidence suggests that small-gauge IV lines (such as 24 gauge) may be maintained more successfully with heparin, whereas larger lines may be maintained with either saline or heparin. Check on policy in your clinical agency.

SKILL 9-4 Administering an IV Push Bolus of Medication: Medication Lock in Place

PREPARATION

1. Check the order.
2. Calculate and check the medication dosage and concentration.
3. Verify the identity of the child and explain the procedure to the child and parents.

EQUIPMENT AND SUPPLIES

- Alcohol swabs
- Two 1- to 2-mL syringes filled with normal saline with 19- to 25-gauge needles or a needleless system
- Syringe filled with 1 mL of heparin flush solution (10 units/mL) or sterile normal saline
- Medication in syringe covered with a 19- to 25-gauge needle

PROCEDURE *Clean Gloves*

1. Don gloves.
2. Clean the catheter cap with alcohol. Unclamp the medication lock.

3. Pierce the catheter cap with a normal saline-filled syringe.

4. Flush the line with 2 mL of normal saline to check patency.

5. Remove the syringe and needle.

6. Insert the medication syringe through the catheter cap and give the medication according to the prescriber's orders. Check a medication resource book or call your hospital pharmacy to determine the rate of administration. When all of the medication has been administered, remove the syringe.

7. Flush the line with the 2 mL of normal saline, followed by the heparin flush solution if the latter is used. Clamp and secure the medication line.

8. Discard the equipment in a puncture-proof container according to standard precaution recommendations.

9. Document the procedure and the child's response.

Intravenous Infusion

The amount of fluid to be administered to a child is based on the child's weight and pathophysiologic state. It is recommended that fluids be given to the infant or child through an infusion pump (Figure 9-4), since this device allows for a more accurate setting of flow rates than gravity does. Maintenance fluid requirements are based on the child's weight (see Table 9-1).

Pumps

An infusion pump can be used to control the administration of small volumes of fluid, blood, medication, and total parenteral nutrition. A smaller syringe pump (Figure 9-5) can be attached directly to the lowest port on the IV tubing for immediate infusion of medication.

It is important to be familiar with the type of infusion pump used at your institution. Be sure to set controls for both the amount of fluid to be infused and the rate of infusion. Check the pump frequently to be certain it is programmed and working correctly.

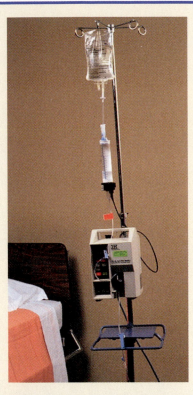

Figure 9-4 *IV setup with infusion pump.*

TABLE 9-1	Pediatric Maintenance Fluid Requirements
Weight (kg)	**Fluid Requirements**
0–10	100 mL/kg/24 hr
10–20	1000 mL + 50 mL/kg/24 hr for each kg between 11 and 20
20–70	1500 mL + 20 mL/kg/24 hr for each kg between 21 and 70
Over 70	2500 mL/24 hr (adult requirement)

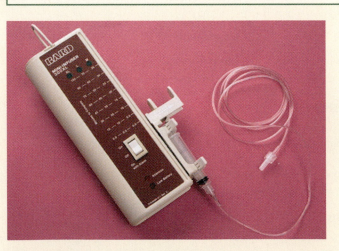

Figure 9-5 *Syringe pump.*

SKILL 9-5 Administering IV Fluids

PREPARATION

1. Check the fluid order for type of IV fluid and infusion rate. Compare with the fluid needs of the child (see your textbook for calculation of children's maintenance and replacement fluids).
2. Gather supplies.
3. Verify the identity of the child and explain the procedure to the child and parent.

EQUIPMENT AND SUPPLIES

- Intravenous fluid
- Tubing
- Infusion pump
- Tape and labels

PROCEDURE *Clean Gloves*

1. Check the bag or bottle for leaks, expiration date, impurities, or color changes.
2. Open the tubing package. Make sure that the tubing is clamped off.
3. Remove the protective covering from the insertion piece (spike). Place the insertion piece into the entry port of the bag or bottle. Invert the bag or bottle and hang it on a pole.
4. Pinch the drip chamber (it should be no more than one half to three fourths full). Direct the distal end of the tubing into a clean receptacle, maintaining sterility of the end. Open the clamp and let the fluid run through the length of the tubing. Tap the tubing at each port to remove any trapped air.
5. Close the clamp, recap the sterile end, and check the entire length of tubing for air bubbles. The tubing is now primed and ready for use.
6. If a volume control chamber (Soluset or Metriset) is used, first attach it to the bag or bottle. Close the clamp that is closest to the fluid and the one that is distal to the chamber. Open the top clamp.
7. Let about 50 mL into the chamber and then close the clamp. Pinch the drip chamber as in step 4. Open the distal clamp, and continue to purge the tubing (as described in step 5).
8. If you are using a pump, check the manufacturer's guidelines for purging the tubing.
9. Mark the bottle or bag with a label and tape that lists the child's identifying information, type of infusion, flow rate, and date and time of preparation.
10. Bring the primed intravenous infusion to the child.
11. Don gloves.
12. Check the IV site carefully for leakage, redness, pallor, swelling, and pain.
13. If replacing a bag that is finished, clamp the tubing on the venous line and on the existing tubing before removing the old tubing.
14. Remove the cover on the end of the IV tubing, maintaining sterility of the tip.
15. Place the tip of the new primed tubing into the existing IV line.
16. Unclamp the IV line and the tubing and begin the flow of fluid.
17. Check the site carefully for leakage, redness, pallor, swelling, and pain as the infusion begins. Repeat assessments according to agency policy.
18. Document the application of a new bag and update the intake of the child considering the bag that has infused.

Guidelines for Infusion of IV Fluids

Rules for determining flow rate for instilling IV fluids via gravity are based on the drip factor of the IV tubing being used.

Microdrip Tubing

Manufacturer	Drops/mL
All major manufacturers	60 drops (gtt) = 1 mL

Formula

mL/hr = gtt/min

Example

1000 mL/8 hr = 125 mL/hr = 125 gtt/min

Macrodrip Tubing

Manufacturer	Drops/mL
Abbot	15 gtt = 1 mL
Baxter	10 gtt = 1 mL

Formula

Total volume × Drop factor/Infusion time in minutes = Drops/minute

Example

1000 mL × 10 (Baxter)/8 hr (480 min) = 21 gtt/min

Blood Administration

To safely administer blood or blood products to the infant or child, be aware of the protocols followed at your agency. Check to be sure that an informed consent for administration is present in the chart. Since hypersensitivity reactions can occur and other side effects can be severe, administration of blood is approached with many nursing cautions. Be sure to take vital signs and monitor the child closely. Follow instructions from the blood bank and other resources for correct administration of blood products, such as frozen plasma, cryoprecipitate, and clotting factors.

SKILL 9-6 Administering Blood or Blood Products

NURSING ALERT

Blood is administered according to the physician's orders. However, a bag should never remain hanging longer than 4 hours. Do not use the blood line for any other infusions. If a medication must be administered by that line, turn off the infusion, flush the line with normal saline, administer the medication, flush the line again with normal saline, and then restart the blood infusion.

PREPARATION

1. Identify the bag to be used, and compare it with the requisition (type, Rh factor, patient number, blood donor number) and the child's identification bracelet. Do this step with another licensed nurse at the bedside. Both nurses are responsible for signing the slips as the transfusers.
   RATIONALE: *Administration of blood has serious implications for injury to the patient. Having two nurses check minimizes the opportunity for error.*

2. Check the blood for any bubbles, dark areas, or sediment.
   RATIONALE: *These discolorations can indicate that the blood is old or has not been properly maintained.*

3. Explain the procedure to the child and parents. Ask the child or family about previous transfusions, especially any history of allergic reactions.

4. Take the child's vital signs, including pulse, respiratory rate, temperature, and blood pressure.
   RATIONALE: *Baseline vital signs may be useful for comparison later in the procedure.*

5. When estimating preparation time, keep in mind that blood must be hung within 20 to 30 minutes after being removed from the blood bank refrigerator. For trauma patients who need

massive transfusions, the bag should be warmed to 37°C (99°F) (only an approved blood warmer should be used).

6. Use the correct tubing for the blood product being administered. A Y blood administration set is preferred. If a Y setup is used, hang normal saline at the extra connector.

EQUIPMENT AND SUPPLIES

- Blood product
- Blood warmer if needed
- Blood filter if needed
- Y tubing and bag of normal saline
- Normal saline flush solution
- Sterile needle or needleless system
- Intravenous line in place with 18-gauge needle or larger

PROCEDURE *Clean or Sterile Gloves*

1. Don gloves. Attach the blood bag to one end of the Y tubing. Flush the line with normal saline attached to the other side of the Y tubing.

   RATIONALE: *Checking the line for patency and using normal saline to prevent incompatibilities contribute to safe infusion.*

2. Clamp off the tubing, keeping the distal end covered.

3. Disconnect it, covering the hub with a sterile needle or needleless system to keep it sterile. Flush the child's IV line with normal saline to ensure its patency.

4. Attach the blood tubing.

5. Slowly open the clamp on the tubing, adjusting the flow with the roller. Start the transfusion slowly. Instruct the child and/or parent to report any reactions immediately.

6. The flow rate may be increased if no reaction is noted.

   RATIONALE: *Most reactions occur within 20 minutes.*

7. Closely monitor the child's vital signs and response. Vital signs should be taken every 5 minutes for the first 15 minutes, every 15 minutes during the first hour, then hourly until the transfusion is complete (or follow your hospital's protocol).

8. If the child develops any sign of a transfusion reaction (Table 9-2), stop the transfusion, change the IV to normal saline, and notify the physician immediately.

> ### HOME CARE CONSIDERATIONS
>
> When a child receives a transfusion of blood or blood products, administration of immunizations must be delayed for several months afterward. Live vaccines such as measles and varicella immunizations are particularly ineffective following blood transfusions. Be sure to let parents know and provide in writing the type of product used (whole blood, packed red cells, frozen plasma, etc.), and the date of the infusion. Instruct them to take this with them when they next visit their regular care provider so that adaptations in the immunization schedule may be implemented if needed.

TABLE 9-2	Transfusion Reactions	
Type of Reaction	**Cause**	**Description**
Allergic	Caused by immune response to protein in blood	Signs and symptoms may include rash, itching, urticaria, wheezing, laryngospasm, edema, and/or anaphylaxis
Febrile or septic	Usually a result of contamination of blood; may also be caused by idiopathic conditions	Signs and symptoms include chills, fever, headache, decreased blood pressure, nausea and/or vomiting, and leg or back pain
Hemolytic	Caused by incompatibility of child's blood with donor blood, history of multiple transfusions, or infusion with a solution containing dextrose or other additives	Signs and symptoms include anxiety or restlessness, fever, chills, chest pain, cyanosis, change in vital signs with increased heart and respiratory rates or with decreased blood pressure and/or hematuria; can progress to shock and anuria if not treated promptly
Circulatory overload	Results from infusion of excessive amounts of fluid or too rapid administration	Signs and symptoms include labored breathing, chest or lower back pain, productive cough with rales heard on auscultation, and distended neck veins; central venous pressure may increase

9. After the administration of blood, flush the line with normal saline and connect the IV fluid ordered by the physician. Place the used blood bag and tubing in a plastic bag, seal it, and return it to the blood bank with copies of the transfusion information sheet.
   RATIONALE: *This is a method of verification of the blood use and the patient data.*

10. Document blood administration, vital signs, responses, and interventions.

SKILL 9-7 Total Parenteral Nutrition

HOME CARE CONSIDERATIONS

Total parenteral nutrition is increasingly administered in the home setting. It may run continuously or be started at night to enable the child needing extra dietary supplementation to have enhanced intake while sleeping. Be sure that parents understand infusion techniques, care of the line, and where to call with questions. Visit the home to be sure the setting can facilitate TPN treatment.

Total parenteral nutrition (TPN) is the administration of a nutritionally complete formula into a large central vein (see Figure 9-6). TPN is used for children who cannot tolerate gastrointestinal feeding. Children with disorders such as chronic intestinal obstruction, short bowel syndrome, chronic diarrhea, or tumors may require TPN.

Hyperalimentation solutions (TPN as well as lipid emulsions) are delivered by separate pumps and connector tubes. The child who is receiving TPN has a central venous catheter in place (see following skill). Solutions and tubes need to be changed every 24 hours using strict aseptic technique. Tips and connecting points need to be sterile. Nursing responsibilities when caring for a child receiving TPN are outlined in Table 9-3.

TABLE 9-3	Caring for the Child Receiving TPN

- Monitor intake and output. Changes may indicate fluid and electrolyte disturbances.
- Weigh the child daily.
- Assess the IV site. Watch for signs of redness, irritation, or infection. Change the dressing according to hospital protocol (see the procedure for managing a central venous catheter site in this chapter).
- Use the infusion site only for TPN solutions or keep the line open with normal saline. Do not use the line for medications or other infusions.
- Make sure to set each pump correctly, noting the volume and rate of each infusion.
- Check laboratory values, especially glucose, minerals, electrolytes, liver function (bilirubin, alkaline phosphatase), proteins, and triglycerides.
- Note any change in glucose levels:
  1. During the first few days, the high concentration of glucose administration may lead to hyperglycemia. Inform the physician of high blood glucose levels. Insulin may be needed to help the body adjust to the formula.
  2. If hyperalimentation is discontinued abruptly, the child may become hypoglycemic. Be aware of the signs and symptoms of hypoglycemia (see your textbook for a full description). Notify the physician if the child's blood glucose level is low.

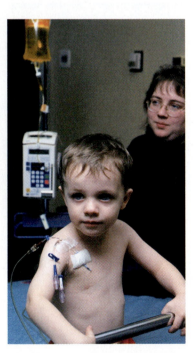

Figure 9-6 *This child is receiving TPN.*

Central Venous Catheters

A central venous catheter is surgically placed when long-term IV access is needed, such as for TPN, administration of antibiotics, or chemotherapy. Usually the subclavian vein is accessed and the catheter is threaded into the right atrium.

The most common catheter used for children is the Broviac™ catheter (Figure 9-7), which can have a single, double, or triple lumen. Other catheters such as the Hickman may be used with older children. Peripherally inserted central catheter lines (PICC lines) are also common in children. Catheter lines require flushing; Broviac™ catheters are flushed once a day, both at home and in the hospital, if they are not accessed for infusions. For flushing, 5 mL of heparin flush solution is used. Consult agency policies for frequency of flushing of these catheters. In addition, the site requires care which is described in the following procedure.

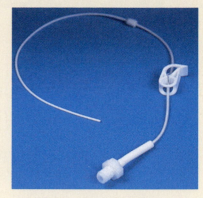

Figure 9-7 *Broviac™ catheter.*

Site Management

The catheter site is covered with a clear occlusive dressing that should be changed under sterile conditions two to three times a week according to agency protocol.

SKILL 9-8 Caring for a Central Venous Catheter Site

PREPARATION

1. Gather necessary supplies.
2. Evaluate the dressing and visible skin at the catheter site.
3. Verify the identity of the child and explain the procedure to the child and parent.
4. Assess the catheter location.

EQUIPMENT AND SUPPLIES

- Peroxide-saturated cotton swabs
- Alcohol swabs
- Chlorhexidine or povidone-iodine swabs
- Central venous catheter kit
- Sterile occlusive dressing

PROCEDURE *Clean and Sterile Gloves (If not using a kit with gloves enclosed), Mask*

1. Open the kit. Don the mask and clean gloves.
2. Remove the current dressing, working from the edges toward the center. Discard the old dressing and gloves.
3. Perform hand hygiene and don the sterile gloves.
4. Clean the catheter site with sterile half-strength peroxide-saturated cotton swabs in an outward circular motion from the point of entry, using one swab for each motion and then changing to a clean one. Clean the area again with alcohol swabs three times, then chlorhexidine or povidone-iodine swabs, using the same technique.
5. Clean the catheter tubing from the exit site to the cap.
6. Let dry. Apply antibacterial ointment around the exit site. Place a small sterile gauze dressing over and under the catheter insertion site. Cover with a sterile occlusive dressing.
7. Write the date, time, and your initials on a piece of tape and place it on the dressing.
8. Document the procedure, the condition of the site, and the child's response.

SKILL 9-9 Accessing a Central Venous Catheter

A central line may be accessed for the drawing of blood samples. The single-syringe method is described here.

PREPARATION

1. Check the physician's order for the blood tests to be done.
   RATIONALE: *It is recommended that the catheter be accessed no more than twice a day to minimize the chance of infection.*
2. Verify the identity of the child and explain the procedure to the child and parent.
3. Locate an assistant to open and close the clamps as necessary and put the blood in tubes while you are flushing the line.

EQUIPMENT AND SUPPLIES

- Sterile 4 × 4 gauze pad
- Chlorhexidine or povidone-iodine solution per agency protocol
- Cotton-tipped swabs
- Appropriate blood collection tubes
- 19-gauge needle for transferring blood to tubes
- Padded clamp (if a clamp is not attached to tubing)

For each port accessed:

- Syringe filled with 5 to 6 mL of normal saline
- Syringe filled with 20 mL of normal saline
- Syringe filled with 2 to 3 mL of heparin flush solution (10 units/mL)
- 5- to 6-mL empty syringe (to draw and discard initial blood)
- Syringes for blood samples
- Luer-lok or Broviac catheter cap

PROCEDURE *Sterile Gloves, Mask*

1. Unpin the catheter from the child's clothes. Remove any tape. Open a sterile 4 × 4 gauze pad to serve as a clean work area. Don sterile gloves. Place the gauze under the catheter connection. If the intravenous solution is infusing, turn it off (Figure 9-8).

2. Clean the connection site with chlorhexidine or povidone-iodine. Use three swabs, and clean for a total of 2 minutes. Let the connection site dry for an additional 20 seconds.

3. Make sure the catheter is clamped. Remove the catheter cap or infusion tubing, maintaining sterility. Flush the catheter with 2 to 5 mL of normal saline to ensure patency. Slowly aspirate 3 to 5 mL of blood (2 mL for infants < 7.5 kg). Clamp the catheter and discard the syringe. Using another 10-mL syringe, aspirate the amount of blood necessary. Remove the blood-filled syringe, and cover with a 19-gauge needle or needleless system. Give that syringe to your assistant to fill the blood collection tubes. Meanwhile, attach the syringe filled with normal saline. Flush the line first with the 20 mL of normal saline, then with the prepared heparin flush solution.

4. Clamp the catheter and remove the flush syringe. Connect the infusion solution, or cover the port with a sterile protector.

5. Secure the catheter to the child's clothing. Remove the gloves and wash your hands.

6. Ensure that blood specimens are labeled properly, kept at proper temperature, and transported to the laboratory.

7. Document the procedure, the condition of the catheter site, and the child's response, and note that the specimens were transported to the laboratory.

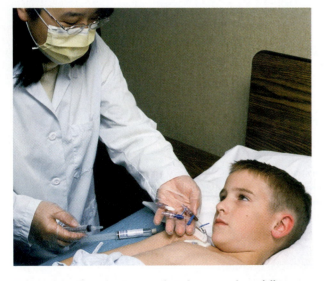

Figure 9-8 *The nurse uses sterile technique and carefully examines the central line to plan access from the proper port.*

SKILL 9-10 Implanted Ports

Implanted ports are used most often for children and adolescents who require long-term venous access. The stainless steel port has a self-sealing rubber septum and is surgically implanted under the skin over a bony prominence, most often the clavicle. The catheter is then inserted into the vein that leads to the right atrium. Entry is gained by piercing the skin directly over the port with a specially designed needle (Figure 9-9). Sterile gloves, mask, and gown are worn when accessing the site. Specially trained nurses may access the site to administer chemotherapy or other medications. Consult agency policy and advanced practice resources for more information about accessing implanted ports.

The Port-a-Cath is used commonly in pediatrics.

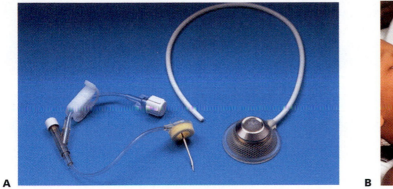
A

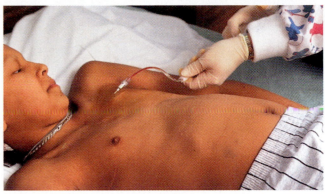
B

Figure 9-9 *A, Huber needle. B, Nurse drawing blood from an adolescent who has an implanted port.*

10

Pain Assessment and Management

CHAPTER OUTLINE

Pain Assessment

Pain is considered the fifth vital sign, and every child has the right to be assessed for pain and receive pain management. The goal of pain assessment is to provide accurate information about the location and intensity of pain and its effects on the child's functioning. Various pain scales have been developed to assess pain in children. Some pain assessment scales rely on the nurse's observation of the child's behavior if the child is nonverbal. Other scales depend on the child's report of pain intensity. For more information, refer to your textbook.

SKILL 10-1 Selected Pediatric Pain Scales

Neonatal Infant Pain Scale (NIPS)

- Use in preterm and term infants up to 6 weeks after birth.
- Observe the infant's facial expression, cry quality, breathing pattern, arm and leg position, and state of arousal (Table 10-1).

TABLE 10-1	Neonatal Infant Pain Scale (NIPS)
Characteristic	**Scoring Criteria**
Facial Expression	
0 = Relaxed muscles	■ Restful face with neutral expression
1 = Grimace	■ Tight facial muscles; furrowed brow, chin, and jaw (Note: At low gestational ages, infants may have no facial expression.)
Cry	
0 = No cry	■ Quiet, not crying
1 = Whimper	■ Mild moaning, intermittent cry
2 = Vigorous cry	■ Loud screaming, rising, shrill, and continuous (Note: Silent cry may be scored if infant is intubated, as indicated by obvious facial movements.)
Breathing Patterns	
0 = Relaxed	■ Relaxed, usual breathing pattern maintained
1 = Change in breathing	■ Change in breathing, irregular, faster than usual, gagging, or holding breath
Arm Movements	
0 = Relaxed/restrained	■ Relaxed, no muscle rigidity, occasional random (with soft restraints) movements of arms
1 = Flexed/extended	■ Tense, straight arms; rigid; or rapid extension and flexion
Leg Movements	
0 = Relaxed/restrained	■ Relaxed, no muscle rigidity, occasional random (with soft restraints) movements of legs
1 = Flexed/extended	■ Tense, straight legs; rigid; or rapid extension and flexion
State of Arousal	
0 = Sleeping/awake	■ Quiet, peaceful, sleeping; or alert and settled
1 = Fussy	■ Alert and restless or thrashing; fussy

Source: Reprinted with permission from Children's Hospital of Eastern Ontario.

FLACC Pain Scale

- This scale is designed to measure acute pain in infants and young children following surgery or while sleeping.
- FLACC is an acronym for the five categories that are assessed: Face, Legs, Activity, Cry, and Consolability (Table 10-2).
- Use until the child is able to self-report pain with another pain scale.

TABLE 10-2 **FLACC Behavioral Pain Assessment Scale**

Categories	Scoring		
	0	**1**	**2**
Face	No particular expression or smile	Occasional grimace or frown; withdrawn, disinterested	Frequent to constant frown, clenched jaw, quivering chin
Legs	Normal position or relaxed	Uneasy, restless, tense	Kicking or legs drawn up
Activity	Lying quietly, normal position, moves easily	Squirming, shifting back and forth, tense	Arched, rigid, or jerking
Cry	No cry (awake or asleep)	Moans or whimpers, occasional complaint	Crying steadily, screams or sobs; frequent complaints
Consolability	Content, relaxed	Reassured by occasional touching, hugging, or being talked to; distractable	Difficult to console or comfort

How to Use the FLACC

In patients who are awake: observe for 1 to 5 minutes or longer. Observe legs and body uncovered. Reposition patient or observe activity. Assess body for tenseness and tone. Initiate consoling interventions if needed.

In patients who are asleep: observe for 5 minutes or longer. Observe body and legs uncovered. If possible, reposition the patient. Touch the body and assess for tenseness and tone.

Face
- Score 0 if the patient has a relaxed face, makes eye contact, shows interest in surroundings.
- Score 1 if the patient has a worried facial expression, with eyebrows lowered, eyes partially closed, cheeks raised, mouth pursed.
- Score 2 if the patient has deep furrows in the forehead, closed eyes, an open mouth, deep lines around nose and lips.

Legs
- Score 0 if the muscle tone and motion in the limbs are normal.
- Score 1 if patient has increased tone, rigidity, or tension; if there is intermittent flexion or extension of the limbs.
- Score 2 if patient has hypertonicity, the legs are pulled tight, there is exaggerated flexion or extension of the limbs, tremors.

Activity
- Score 0 if the patient moves easily and freely, normal activity or restrictions.
- Score 1 if the patient shifts positions, appears hesitant to move, demonstrates guarding, a tense torso, pressure on a body part.
- Score 2 if the patient is in a fixed position, rocking; demonstrates side-to-side head movement or rubbing of a body part.

Cry
- Score 0 if the patient has no cry or moan, awake or asleep.
- Score 1 if the patient has occasional moans, cries, whimpers, sighs.
- Score 2 if the patient has frequent or continuous moans, cries, grunts.

Consolability
- Score 0 if the patient is calm and does not require consoling.
- Score 1 if the patient responds to comfort by touching or talking in 30 seconds to 1 minute.
- Score 2 if the patient requires constant comforting or is inconsolable.

Whenever feasible, behavioral measurement of pain should be used in conjunction with self-report. When self-report is not possible, interpretation of pain behaviors and decisions regarding treatment of pain require careful consideration of the context in which the pain behaviors are observed.

Interpreting the Behavioral Score

Each category is scored on the 0–2 scale, which results in a total score of 0–10.

0 = Relaxed and comfortable	**4–6** = Moderate pain
1–3 = Mild discomfort	**7–10** = Severe discomfort or pain or both

From Merkel, S. I., Voepel-Lewis, T., Shayevitz, J. R., & Malviya, S. (1997). The FLACC: A behavioral scale for scoring postoperative pain in young children. *Pediatric Nursing, 23*(3), 293–297. The FLACC scale was developed by Sandra Merkel, MS, RN, Terri Voepel-Lewis, MS, RN, and Shobha Malviya, MD, at C. S. Mott Children's Hospital, University of Michigan Health System, Ann Arbor, MI. Used with permission.

Oucher Scale

- Use in children between 3 and 7 years of age. Select the scale that matches the child's ethnic background—Caucasian, African American, or Hispanic (Figure 10-1).
- The child selects the face that matches his or her level of pain. The older child can select a number between 0 and 10.

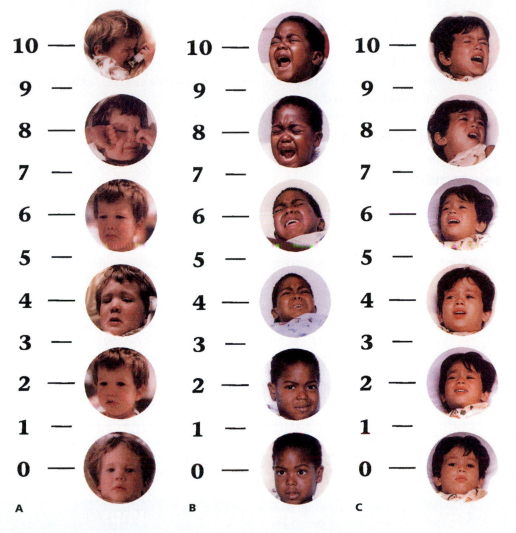

A   B   C

Figure 10-1 *Oucher Scale 3–7 years.* *In the form presented in this book, the Oucher is for educational purposes only and cannot be used for patient care.
A, The Caucasian version of the Oucher, developed and copyrighted by Judith E. Beyer, RN, Ph.D., 1983.
B, The African-American version of the Oucher, developed and copyrighted by Mary J. Denyes, RN, Ph.D., 1990. Cornelia P. Porter, RN, Ph.D., and Charlotta Marshall, RN, MSN, contributed to the development of the scale. *C*, The Hispanic version of the Oucher, developed and copyrighted by Antonia M. Villarruel, RN, Ph.D., and Mary J. Denyes, RN, Ph.D., 1990.

FACES Pain Rating Scale

- Use in children from 3 years through adolescence.
- The child selects the face that is the closest match to the amount of pain felt (Figure 10-2).

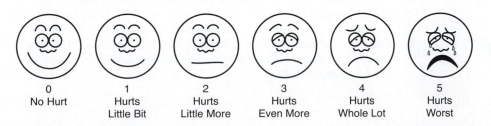

| 0 | 1 | 2 | 3 | 4 | 5 |
| No Hurt | Hurts Little Bit | Hurts Little More | Hurts Even More | Hurts Whole Lot | Hurts Worst |

Figure 10-2 *FACES Pain Rating Scale. After determining that the child has an understanding of number concepts, teach the child how to use the scale. Point to each face and use the words under the picture to describe the amount of pain the child feels. Then ask the child to select the face that comes closest to the amount of pain felt.*
From Hockenberry, M. J.: *Wong's Essentials of Pediatric Nursing*, ed. 7, St. Louis, 2005, Mosby, p. 1301.
Copyrighted by Mosby, Inc. Reprinted by permission.

Numeric Pain Scale

- Use in children from 9 years to adult.
- Ask the child to rate the pain felt on a line with 10 marks, with 1 indicating a little pain and 10 indicating the most pain ever felt (Figure 10-3).

```
|----|----|----|----|----|----|----|----|----|----|
0    1    2    3    4    5    6    7    8    9    10
```

Figure 10-3 *Numeric pain scale.*

PREPARATION

1. Select the pain scale appropriate for the age, cooperation, and communication ability of the child.
2. Explain the procedure to the child and parents.
3. Teach the cooperative and communicative child how to use the pain scale.

EQUIPMENT AND SUPPLIES

Copy of the pain scale

PROCEDURE

> **GROWTH AND DEVELOPMENT**
>
> Even newborns and infants feel and remember pain. Children may not complain about pain because they fear the method to relieve pain is worse than the pain.

1. Perform a pain assessment with a child each time you initiate new care and any time an adult would be expected to have pain, such as from an injury, surgery, or illness.
   RATIONALE: *JCAHO requires a pain assessment during outpatient visits and hospital admissions.*
2. When the child is able to verbalize, ask the child to point to the picture or number that matches how the child feels at that moment. Some pain scales have a standardized way to ask the question.
3. If the child has multiple injuries, ask about the pain felt at each site, and then all injuries together.
   RATIONALE: *Assessment of the pain only associated with an individual injury may minimize the overall pain or discomfort the child is feeling.*
4. Repeat the pain assessment after analgesia is given and compare with the earlier pain assessment.
   RATIONALE: *This action determines the effectiveness of the analgesia provided and facilitates individualized pain management.*
5. Document the pain assessment method, score, and time performed.

Special Pain Management Techniques

SKILL 10-2 Administering Patient-Controlled Analgesia (PCA) Pumps

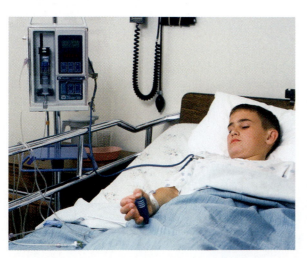

Specially designed pumps can be used to deliver analgesia to individuals for pain control. The pumps use an intravenous line and a syringe with ordered medication locked inside the pump. The pump is programmed so that when the patient pushes a button, a preset analgesic dose is administered. If it is too soon, the pump will not deliver the dose since a lockout interval is programmed into the pump computer by the nurse. In addition, the pump can be set to administer a specific amount of medication at designated time intervals without the child pushing the button. This allows for pain control even during sleep or for young children (Figure 10-4).

Figure 10-4 *This boy was instructed preoperatively in use of the PCA pump. Being able to administer his own analgesia when it is needed offers him a sense of control and contributes to successful pain management.*

PREPARATION

1. When it is assumed that a child will have a PCA after surgery, bring it in before the surgery and explain its use to the child and parents.

   RATIONALE: *This will enhance the child's understanding since he or she is not in pain or immediately postoperative.*

2. Once ordered, check the medication order and compute the maximum 24-hour dose to verify safety.

3. Prepare the tubing and pump according to manufacturer directions.

   RATIONALE: *The PCA tubing needs to be primed with IV fluid and attached with a Y connector to the IV line for the patient.*

EQUIPMENT AND SUPPLIES

- Pump
- Tubing
- IV fluid
- Medication
- Alcohol swabs

PROCEDURE *Clean Gloves*

1. Complete a thorough pain and physical assessment.

   RATIONALE: *Baseline data are used to evaluate pain control effectiveness and any side effects from the medication.*

2. Bring the prepared tubing, pump, and medication to the child.

3. Don gloves.

4. Attach the tubing as directed to the child's IV line.

5. Unlock the pump door and follow protocol for programming the pump delivery.

6. Deliver a loading dose if ordered.

   RATIONALE: *Loading doses begin the medication process and allow pain control to be achieved more rapidly.*

7. Verify that the pump is locked and the key is removed from the room.

   RATIONALE: *Inadvertent entry of unauthorized persons into the pump mechanism must be avoided.*

8. Continue to reassess the child's pain to ensure adequate pain control, and make the needed adjustment to the care plan.

SKILL 10-3 Sedation Monitoring

Sedation is increasingly being used in children since it offers a method of safely performing painful procedures and avoiding trauma to the child. With moderate sedation (formerly called conscious sedation), consciousness is depressed while the child is able to maintain a patent airway and can respond to some verbal commands and to physical stimulation. With deep sedation the child has reflex activity, but is unable to respond to pain or verbal commands (Bindler & Howry, 2005). When sedation will be provided, it is important that the child is properly prepared, monitored during the procedure, and recovered after the procedure is completed.

PREPARATION

1. Inform the child (if old enough to understand) and parents. Ensure that informed consent is obtained.

2. Obtain assessment data outlined in Table 10-3.

3. Evaluate recent food and fluid intake.

   RATIONALE: *Desired time for the child to be NPO for foods is 8 hours, and for fluids 4 to 6 hours. Time intervals are shorter for infants.*

4. Verify sedation orders.

TABLE 10-3	Assessments Prior to Sedation

History	Physical Examination
Age	Vital signs
Health history including diseases, hospitalizations, family history, review of systems	Weight and height
	Physical status by trained anesthetist or anesthesiologist
Allergies	Physical examination
Current medications	Focused airway assessment
Prior complications with sedation	Time since last food and fluid intake

Source: Adapted from Bindler, R. M., & Howry, L. B. (2005). *Pediatric Drug Guide with nursing implications.* Upper Saddle River, NJ: Prentice Hall Health.

EQUIPMENT AND SUPPLIES

- Have drugs to be used prepared and available (Table 10-4). Prepare emergency drugs. Have opioid and benzodiazepine reversal agents (naloxone, flumazenil) available if these medications are used for sedation.

    RATIONALE: *The practitioner using sedation must be trained in use of the medication and in airway management. An additional support person must be present to monitor the child. All personnel present should be trained in advanced life support in emergency situations.*

- Emergency equipment must be immediately available, including oxygen, suction, oral and nasal airways, resuscitation bag and mask, laryngoscope, endotracheal tube, pulse oximeter, and cardiopulmonary monitor.
- Make sure syringes and IV lines and fluids are available.
- Have respiratory suction present and functional.

PROCEDURE *Clean and Sterile Gloves*

During Procedure

1. Record all drugs administered, doses, and times.
2. Monitor oxygen saturation and heart rate continuously.
3. Assess level of sedation, airway patency, respiration, and blood pressure throughout the procedure.
4. Record all assessments on flow sheet according to facility policy.
5. Check procedural immobilizer and head position throughout the procedure.

After Procedure

1. Perform assessments and monitoring while keeping suction and emergency services available.
2. Take vital signs and complete other monitoring every 5 minutes until the patient is awake and then every 15 minutes until stable and discharged.

CLINICAL TIP

Discharge Criteria from Unit after Sedation

- Child has satisfactory and stable cardiovascular function and airway patency.
- Child is easily arousable, with protective reflexes intact.
- Child has adequate hydration.
- Child sits up unassisted if old enough to do so.
- If child is very young or has a disability, discharge state is same as admission state.

Source: Adapted from Bindler, R. M., & Howry, L. B. (2005). *Pediatric Drug Guide with nursing implications* (p. 49). Upper Saddle River, NJ: Prentice Hall Health.

TABLE 10-4	Common Medications Used for Sedation

- Benzodiazepines: diazepam (Valium), midazolam (Versed), and lorazepam (Ativan)
- Hypnotics or barbiturates: thiopental, pentobarbital
- Ketamine
- Propofol (Diprivan)
- Analgesics: fentanyl, alfentanil

Source: Data from Proudfoot, J. (2002). Pediatric procedural sedation and analgesia (PSA): Keeping it simple and safe. *Pediatric Emergency Medicine Reports, 7*(2), 1–2.

SKILL 10-4 Local Pain Blocks

Local pain blocks are increasingly being inserted during surgery or other procedures to offer local pain control. Commonly, microtubing is inserted into a site such as the epidural space or popliteal area, wrapped securely, and attached to an infusion pump with pain medication (Figure 10-5A and B). Local pain blocks allow the child to be alert and interactive while achieving excellent pain control.

PREPARATION

1. Have an infusion pump ready when the child may return from surgery with a local block.
2. Review the child's operative and post-anesthesia records, and the medication noted on the infusion bag.

EQUIPMENT AND SUPPLIES

- Medication and pain assessment records
- Infusion pump

PROCEDURE

1. Perform pain assessment and complete vital signs and level of consciousness.
   RATIONALE: *Baseline data will be needed for future comparison.*
2. Observe the wrapped local block site. Evaluate for swelling, redness, pallor, or leaking of solution onto the bandage.
3. Monitor the infusion and maintain at the ordered infusion rate.
4. Continue to monitor regularly according to agency policy.
5. When the block is to be discontinued by the physician, provide sterile gloves, gauze pads, and tape.
6. Monitor the site several times daily until removed for drainage or discharge.
   RATIONALE: *Continued monitoring assists in identifying infection.*

SAFETY PRECAUTIONS

The dressing around a local pain block insertion site should NOT be removed to check the site. This could inadvertently dislodge the catheter. Check the skin that is visible and the dressing for drainage, but do not remove the dressing without specific physician orders.

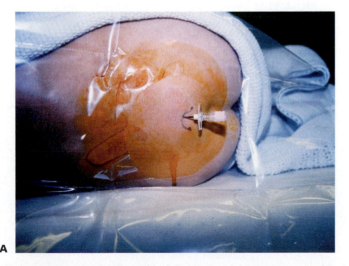
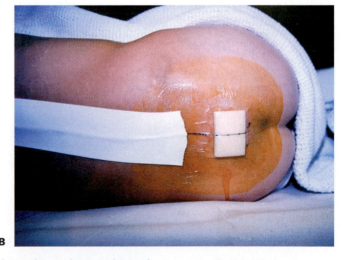

A   B

Figure 10-5 *A, Epidural pain block being placed during surgery, and B, taped into place and wrapped securely.*
Courtesy of Shriners Hospital for Children, Spokane, WA.

11

Cardiorespiratory Care

Administration of Oxygen

When administering oxygen, the concentration ordered and the age of the child are important. Humidification is often necessary to prevent nasal passages from drying out. Because oxygen is combustible, certain precautions must be taken during its use.

Oxygen Delivery Systems

Masks

The size of the mask is important when administering oxygen. The mask should extend from the bridge of the nose to the cleft of the chin. It should fit snugly on the face but put no pressure on the eyes to avoid stimulating a vagal response.
The following types of masks are available:

- The simple face mask (Figure 11-1) can deliver from 30% to 60% oxygen when a flow rate of 6 to 10 L/min is used and a tight seal is maintained on the face.

- The nonrebreather mask (Figure 11-2) has a reservoir bag attached to a simple face mask to deliver higher concentrations of oxygen, from 60% to 90% with a flow of 12 to 15 L/min, when a tight seal is maintained on the face.

Nasal Cannula

A nasal cannula is used to deliver low-flow, low-concentration oxygen. It does not provide humidified oxygen. A flow rate set higher than 6 L/min will irritate the nasopharynx without appreciably improving the child's oxygenation. The nasal cannula can deliver up to 44% oxygen with a flow rate of 1 to 6 L/min.

The prongs of the cannula are placed in the anterior nares, and the elastic band is placed around the child's head (Figure 11-3). Infants, preschoolers, and school-age children usually tolerate the cannula. Toddlers will usually pull the cannula off their face. A face mask or blow-by tubing is often a more appropriate method of oxygen administration for this age group.

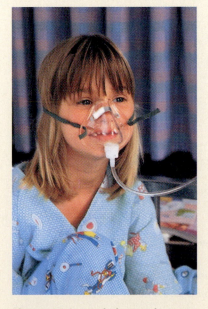

Figure 11-1 *Simple face mask.*

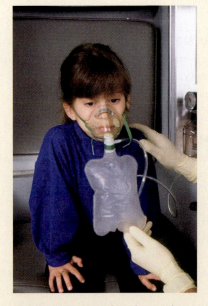

Figure 11-2 *Nonrebreather mask.*

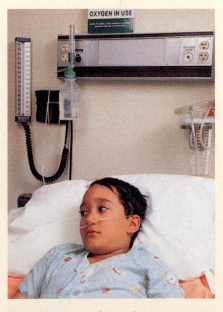

Figure 11-3 *Nasal cannula.*

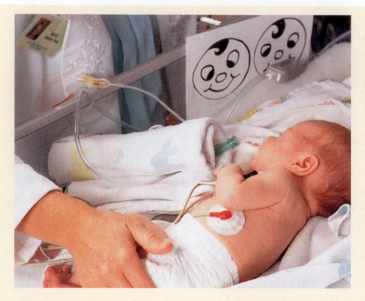

Figure 11-4 *Blow-by cannula.*

Tent

An oxygen tent, in theory, allows for delivery of 50% humidified oxygen, but in practice only 30% humidified oxygen can be achieved. Concentration should be determined with an oxygen analyzer. To avoid air leakage, secure the edges of the tent with blankets.

Access to and visual assessment of the child are difficult when an oxygen tent is used. The child may feel confined, isolated from his or her parents, or claustrophobic when in the tent. The child may respond more favorably to using the mask when awake and the tent while asleep.

Blow-By Cannula

A blow-by cannula may be either a narrow oxygen catheter with small perforations through which oxygen can flow or corrugated oxygen tubing. This device is used when the child will not tolerate other means of oxygen therapy and when low oxygen concentrations with humidification are needed. The concentration of oxygen delivered varies according to the flow rate and proximity to the face. The parent can hold the child in his or her lap and direct the tubing toward the child's face, moving it as the child moves. This technique reduces the child's anxiety and facilitates parental involvement in care. In the intensive care unit (ICU), the blow-by method can be used for young infants (Figure 11-4).

SKILL 11-1 Using Oxygen Delivery Systems

SAFETY PRECAUTIONS

- "Oxygen in Use" signs should be posted at the child's doorway and at the bedside.
- Make sure that matches and lighters are not used in the area.
- Use only hospital-approved electrical equipment.
- Do not use flammable or volatile solutions in the child's room.

PREPARATION

1. Review the physician order for the oxygen delivery system.
2. Verify the identity of the child and explain the procedure to the child and parents.
3. Attach a sterile water-filled container to the oxygen or flow meter with a connecting tube.
4. Inform the child and parent about the need for oxygen, how it will be provided, and how they can assist with the procedure.

EQUIPMENT AND SUPPLIES

- Oxygen canister or wall outlet, tubing, and flow meter
- Oxygen delivery system
- Sterile water-filled container
- Oximeter

PROCEDURE

1. Perform a baseline assessment of vital signs, color, respiratory effort, pulse oximetry reading, and level of consciousness.
   RATIONALE: *The baseline assessment provides a comparison to measure the effectiveness of oxygen therapy.*
2. Turn on oxygen to the ordered flow rate.
3. Place the oxygen delivery device on the child's face. If the child resists the device, check the fit, and try to improve the child's comfort.
4. When an oxygen tent is used, secure the edges to prevent oxygen leakage.
5. Monitor the child's response to the therapy with ongoing assessments compared to baseline.
6. Report and document the child's condition and changes related to oxygen therapy.

Cardiorespiratory Monitoring

SKILL 11-2 Oxygen Saturation: Pulse Oximetry

Pulse oximetry is a simple noninvasive method to measure the percentage of hemoglobin that is available to transport oxygen in the blood by emitting red and infrared light over a pulsating vascular bed and measuring the intensity of light transmitted through the tissue. Hemoglobin absorbs differing amounts of red and infrared light, depending upon how much it is oxygenated (Galley, 2005). An estimate of hemoglobin saturation is calculated (SpO_2, the percentage of hemoglobin that is capable of transporting oxygen).

PREPARATION

1. Verify the identity of the child.

2. Explain the procedure to the child and parent and why it is needed. Inform the child that pulse oximetry is a pain-free method of monitoring the oxygen level in the blood.

3. Select the appropriate sensor size for the child, either infant or pediatric sizes. Size is determined by the size of the child and/or the placement site.

4. Set the oximeter parameters for alarms according to physician directions or agency policy.

EQUIPMENT AND SUPPLIES

- Pulse oximeter
- Appropriate-size sensor

PROCEDURE

1. Perform a baseline assessment before attaching the sensor. Check respiratory status, including heart rate, respiratory rate, skin color, and respiratory effort.

2. Place the sensor on the fingertip over the nail, on the toe over the nail, or on the earlobe (Figure 11-5A and B). It should be approximately at heart level.
   RATIONALE: *The earlobe is used when the child has poor perfusion. This is considered a central location, especially since a large percentage of the blood goes to the head and brain.*

3. Position the sensor with the cord leading toward the patient. Secure the cord to the patient to stabilize the sensor for more reliable readings.

4. Turn on the oximeter. Attach the sensor to the machine. Watch for a readout of the pulse rate and oxygen saturation level.

> ### CLINICAL TIP
>
> To obtain the most accurate pulse oximetry reading, make sure the site of measurement is clean and dry and has minimal movement. To avoid interference of light being transmitted to the vascular bed, no nail polish should be on the finger where the probe is placed. Blue, green, black, or brown nail polish may lead to a low SpO_2 reading. Sunlight and other bright overhead lighting can also falsely increase the oxygen saturation reading (Galley, 2005; Popovich, Richiuso, & Danek, 2004).

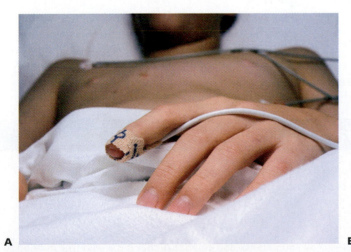
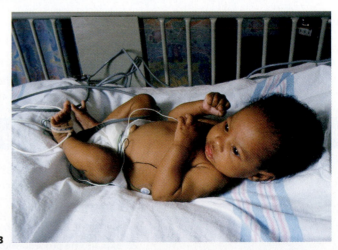

Figure 11-5 *A, Pulse oximeter on finger and B, on foot.*

5. Leave the oximeter on for continuous readouts. If frequent but noncontinuous monitoring is ordered, leave the sensor on the child but disconnect it from the machine.
   RATIONALE: *Disconnecting the machine allows the child freedom to move and feel less confined.*

6. If the sensor is removed, place it on the plastic backing for further use. This maintains the adhesive so the sensor can be reused.

7. Remove the sensor from the extremity at least every 2 hours to check the condition of the skin.

SKILL 11-3 Cardiorespiratory or Apnea Monitor

The standard cardiorespiratory monitor measures heart rate and respiratory rate when continuous assessments of the heart and respiratory rates are required. An apnea monitor is used to monitor for abnormal or irregular breathing in infants.

PREPARATION

1. Verify the identity of the child. Explain the procedure to the child and parents, informing them that this is a pain-free method to monitor the child's condition.

2. The high and low limits are set according to the age of the child and the underlying condition. Usually a 15- to 20-second period of apnea will set off the alarm.

EQUIPMENT AND SUPPLIES

- Cardiorespiratory monitor
- Electrodes and straps to hold them in place
- Alcohol swabs

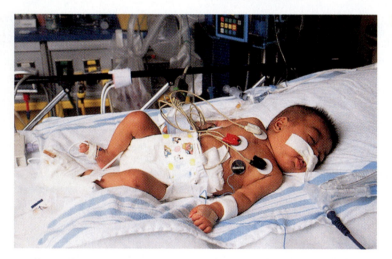

Figure 11-6 *Placement of cardiorespiratory monitor electrodes.*

PROCEDURE

1. Use alcohol swabs to clean the skin areas where the leads will be applied, and allow the skin to dry.
   RATIONALE: *Cleaning the skin will remove oils so the adhesive pads holding the electrodes have better adherence.*

2. Place the electrodes on the child's chest: one on the right side, one on the left, and one (ground) on the lateral side of the abdomen (Figure 11-6).

3. If the monitor alarm sounds, check the child immediately. Assess breathing and heart rate.

4. If the child is not breathing, stimulate the child, reposition the airway, and, if there is no response, initiate cardiopulmonary resuscitation (CPR) and call a code (see Skill 11-18).

5. If the child is not in distress, silence the alarm, check the connections and leads, and reset the alarm.
   RATIONALE: *Leads frequently become disconnected as the child moves and an alarm is triggered.*

6. Document the alarm, the nursing action, and the child's condition.

SKILL 11-4 Placement of Electrocardiogram Electrodes

The electrocardiogram (ECG) is a graphic representation of the electricity produced by the heart muscle. Twelve leads are used to provide the optimal recording.

PREPARATION

1. Verify the identity of the child.

2. Explain the procedure to the child and parents, and emphasize that it is a pain-free method to assess the heart. Discuss the need for the child to remain still during the actual ECG.

EQUIPMENT AND SUPPLIES

- Electrocardiogram recorder
- Patches with leads (or suction cups with conductive gel)
- Alcohol swabs

PROCEDURE

1. Use alcohol swabs to clean the sites where the leads will be placed.

2. Electrodes are placed both on the chest and on the limbs in the locations described in Table 11-1.
   RATIONALE: *Correct placement of the electrodes is important to ensure that the electrical impulses are accurately recorded.*

3. Turn on the electrocardiogram recorder and collect the tracing.

4. When completed, remove the electrodes and remove any conductive gel with moistened gauze pads.

5. Label the tracing and place it in the designated section of the child's medical record.

TABLE 11-1	Placement of Electrocardiogram Electrodes
Chest electrodes	V_1C fourth intercostal space to right of sternum V_2C fourth intercostal space to left of sternum V_3C midway between V_2 and V_4 V_4C fifth left intercostal space at midclavicular line V_5C fifth left intercostal space at anterior axillary line (midway between V_4 and V_6) V_6C fifth left intercostal space at midaxillary line
Limb electrodes	One on each upper extremity slightly above the wrists One on each lower extremity just above the ankles

SKILL 11-5 Peak Expiratory Flow Rate (PEFR) Monitoring

Peak expiratory flow rate meters are often recommended for home use to monitor pulmonary function in children with respiratory conditions such as asthma. The child's personal best average reading is determined by using the PEFR meter frequently over a 2- to 3-week period at several times of the day when the child's asthma is optimally treated (Radeos & Camargo, 2004). This personal best average rate may then be used for comparison when the child has signs of breathing difficulty.

PREPARATION

1. Verify the identity of the child. Explain the procedure to the child and parents and the reasons for its use.

2. The indicator on the peak flow rate meter is placed at the bottom of the numbered scale.

3. The peak flow meter is then set to reflect the child's personal best score and "zones" indicating different levels of expiratory capacity (Table 11-2). These zones are used to guide the action plan for the child's medication management and adjustment.

CLINICAL TIP

Peak expiratory flow rates (PEFR) vary by age, sex, and height. Children under 6 years of age may not have the coordination to use the PEFR meter. The leg length to thoracic cavity ratio helps explain the variability in PEFR to height. PEFR is also believed to vary by race. Black males have lower spirometry readings than whites of European descent, possibly due to differences in the leg length to thoracic cavity ratio. Care must be taken in applying formulas for PEFR to all races when attempting to determine the severity of airway compromise (Radeos & Camargo, 2004).

TABLE 11-2	Assessing Peak Expiratory Flow Rate (PEFR)		

	Zone	PEFR (Best or Predicted for Age)	Action
	Green	80%–100%	Continue regular management plan.
	Yellow	50%–80%	An episode of asthma may be beginning. Implement action plan provided by physician.
	Red	Less than 50%	Medical Alert: Implement action plan predetermined by physician. Call provider if PEFR does not return to yellow or green zone.

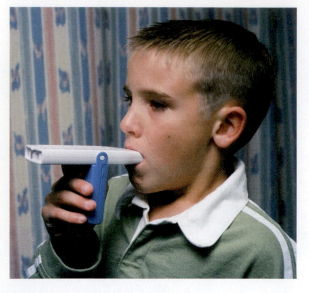

Figure 11-7 *Child with a peak flow meter.*

EQUIPMENT AND SUPPLIES

- Peak flow rate meter
- Notebook to keep a log of PEFR readings

PROCEDURE

1. Have the child stand and place the mouthpiece of the meter in the mouth (Figure 11-7). After taking a deep breath, the child should blow as hard and fast into the meter as he or she can. Read the number achieved.

2. Have the child repeat this procedure two or three more times. Average the numbers from all the readings to derive the PEFR.
   RATIONALE: *The child may need a couple of efforts to get the best reading.*

3. Compare the PEFR with the child's personal best, and interpret the level of respiratory distress and the appropriate intervention.

4. Document the child's PEFR and provide medication if needed.

5. Provide teaching for the parent and child on appropriate technique, recording results, and actions for decreased PEFR readings, if the PEFR monitoring will be performed on a regular basis at home.

SKILL 11-6 Central Venous Pressure Monitoring

Central venous pressure (CVP) or right atrial pressure is the measurement used to assess the filling pressure or preload of the right side of the heart in critically ill children. In a healthy patient, the CVP closely resembles the left atrial pressure and is usually used to predict it. CVP can be monitored using catheters inserted into the right atrium by way of the internal jugular, subclavian, and femoral veins. A manometer filled with intravenous fluid or a transducer attached to the central venous catheter provides the pressure reading. *Central venous line site care is discussed in Chapter 9.*

PREPARATION

1. Verify the identity of the child.

2. Explain the procedure to the child and family. Clarify that the child will not feel any pain or changes.

3. Assemble IV tubing, stopcocks, and high-pressure tubing.

4. Check all IV, stopcock, and manometer or transducer connections to be certain they are tight. If a transducer is used, connect it to the monitor cable.

5. Flush all IV tubing, high-pressure tubing, and stopcocks with heparin IV solution and ensure that the setup is free of air bubbles. Cover each port with a sterile cap.

EQUIPMENT AND SUPPLIES

- IV pole (with transducer bar and transducer cable, if indicated)
- Pressure module
- Infusion pump or pressure bag
- IV tubing—appropriate for CVP monitor equipment
- High-pressure tubing
- Heparin IV solution or IV solution ordered by physician
- T connector
- Level
- 10-mL syringe filled with normal saline

PROCEDURE

1. Verify correct placement of the catheter tip by observation of a change in pressure in different phases of respiration, free aspiration of blood through the catheter, and/or radiologic confirmation.

2. Pressure bag setup: Place the IV bag inside the pressure bag and hang from the IV stand. Inflate the pressure device to 150 mm Hg to 300 mm Hg (and an infusion flow rate of approximately 3 mL/hr) making sure the drip chamber does not fill completely. Confirm the 3 mL/hr infusion rate in the drip chamber.

3. Place the child in a supine position; however, the head of the bed may be elevated.
   RATIONALE: *Inaccurate readings may occur when a patient is turned to the side or repositioned.*

4. Verify that the manometer or transducer is level to the midaxillary or phlebostatic axis.

5. Temporarily stop other IV infusions into the CVP port of the catheter (or as much as the child will tolerate to ensure an accurate reading). Other IVs and medications should infuse into other ports. Always restart any infusions temporarily stopped following the CVP reading.
   RATIONALE: *Infusion of large volumes into the CVP port can falsely elevate the reading.*

6. Manometer reading:
   - The manometer needs to be set to zero at the level of the right atrium (at the fourth intercostal space and midaxillary line when the patient is supine). See Figure 11-8.
   - Take the CVP measurement in the same position each time using a level and the zero point marked on the skin surface with a cross.
   - Check that the catheter is not blocked or kinked and that intravenous fluid runs freely in, and blood flows freely out.
   - Open the three-way stopcock so that the fluid bag fills the manometer tubing (verify that fluid flow is not obstructed and that the cotton wool in the top of the manometer is not blocked or wet).
   - Turn the stopcock to connect the patient to the manometer.
   - The fluid level will drop to the level of the CVP, which is usually recorded in centimeters of water (cm H_2O). The fluid level will be slightly pulsatile, rising and falling slightly with breathing. Record the average reading.

7. Electronic transducers provide a continuous readout of CVP along with a display of the waveform.
   - Connect the transducer to the monitor cable.
   - Level the transducer to the midaxillary (phlebostatic) axis. This levels the transducer with the right atrium and becomes the zero point.
   - Calibrate and set the monitor to zero following guidelines in the monitor manual.
     RATIONALE: *Zeroing the catheter tubing system establishes atmospheric pressure as zero and compensates for the hydrostatic effect of fluid in the catheter tubing system. This zeroing ensures pressures within the vessels or heart chamber are measured.*
   - The CVP reading from an electronic monitor may be reported in mm Hg. The values may be converted to cm H_2O as 10 cm H_2O equals 7.5 mm Hg.

8. Observe and document the CVP reading. If the patient has large ventilatory tidal volumes, note the reading at the end of expiration. The child's normal reading may vary due to anatomic and physiologic variances.

9. Notify the physician of any rapid changes in CVP readings. The CVP measurement may still be in the normal range even with hypovolemia due to venous constriction.

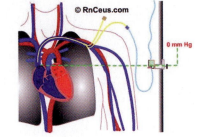

Figure 11-8 *Level for setting the manometer to zero in the midaxillary axis. This position ensures alignment with the right atrium of the heart to give an accurate central venous pressure reading.*
Source: http://www.rnceus.com

CLINICAL TIP

The CVP is often used to make estimates of circulatory function, in particular cardiac function and blood volume. The normal pediatric CVP value is 2 to 6 mm Hg. A high pediatric CVP value is greater than 12 to 18 mm Hg. A low CVP value suggests hypovolemia or decreased venous return. A high CVP value may indicate overhydration, increased venous return, or right-sided cardiac failure.

SKILL 11-7 Arterial Pressure Monitoring

Arterial pressure monitoring allows continuous monitoring of vascular pressures. This type of monitoring is performed when rapid fluctuations in arterial pressure may occur and signal poor perfusion that could precede or accompany the development of a life-threatening crisis. Sites available for arterial pressure monitoring include the radial, axillary, femoral, posterior tibial, and dorsalis pedis arteries.

PREPARATION

1. Verify the child's identity. Explain the procedure to the child and family and the nursing care that will be provided. Describe the activity restrictions that are important to protect the arterial line.

2. Set up and calibrate the pressure monitoring system prior to insertion of the arterial catheter.

EQUIPMENT AND SUPPLIES

- Arterial line placement set
- High-pressure tubing; standard pump tubing may be utilized in a neonatal intensive care unit (NICU).
- IV solution and pump tubing
- T connector of choice
- Chlorhexidine-based preparation or other approved skin preparation
- Alcohol pads
- IV stand with transducer bar and cable
- Arterial blood pressure module
- Level

PROCEDURE *Sterile Gloves, Gown, Eye Protection*

1. Assist the physician with insertion of the arterial line.

2. Maintain the arterial line and provide site care according to hospital guidelines. Patency of the catheter should be maintained with a continuous infusion of flush solution ordered by the physician or per agency policy.

3. Closely observe the extremity distal to the arterial line for temperature, color, pulsation, and capillary refill. Doppler may be used for pulses that are difficult to palpate. Observe for potential complications of arterial cannulation, such as infection and thrombosis with distal ischemia. Assess and document every 4 hours or according to agency policy.

4. Restrict patient activities according to unit protocols and/or physician orders.

5. When attaching the pressure monitoring device to the arterial catheter, every connection should be locked with a Luer-Lok for safety.
   RATIONALE: *A disconnection could mean sudden hemorrhage from the arterial cannulation and could be fatal.*

6. The transducer should be positioned level with the heart, using the level to set the transducer position at the level of the fourth intercostal space at the midclavicular line and midaxillary line. Refer to the monitor manual for guidance as necessary.

7. Ensure that the monitoring device is properly set to zero when the transducer is in the appropriate position. Verify or reset the monitoring device to zero every shift, when the transducer or the patient's position changes, or when readings are questionable.

8. Check the pressure waveform on the monitor to make certain the catheter is patent and functional. A crisp waveform should appear. If dampened, the arterial reading is not accurate.

9. Obtain an auscultated blood pressure at least every shift using the same limb as the arterial catheter, unless contraindicated. Note the correlation between the arterial pressure and the auscultated blood pressure. Intra-arterial measurements are expected to be slightly higher than the auscultated blood pressure since the resistance of distal vessels is higher, and the distance is slightly further.

10. Document the arterial pressure readings, pulsation waveform, auscultated blood pressure, and the limb temperature, capillary refill, and color.

Artificial Airways

SKILL 11-8 Assisting with Oropharyngeal Airway Insertion

The oropharyngeal airway is commonly used to maintain an airway in children who are unconscious. Pediatric sizes range from 4 to 10 centimeters in length. The airway must be the correct size. The oropharyngeal airway is designed to keep the tongue of an unconscious child from falling into the posterior pharynx (Figure 11-9). An oropharyngeal airway is usually inserted by the physician.

PREPARATION

1. Verify the identity of the child. Explain the procedure to the parents (the child is usually unconscious or not fully responsive when an oral airway is inserted).

2. Select the proper size. To determine the proper size oral airway for the child, place an airway alongside the child's face with the bite block parallel to the hard palate and the flange at the level of the central incisors. The distal end of the airway should reach the angle of the jaw (Figure 11-10). Select the airway that is the best fit for the child.
   RATIONALE: *If the airway is too large, it can obstruct the larynx. If it is too small, it will push the tongue into the posterior pharynx, causing it to obstruct the airway.*

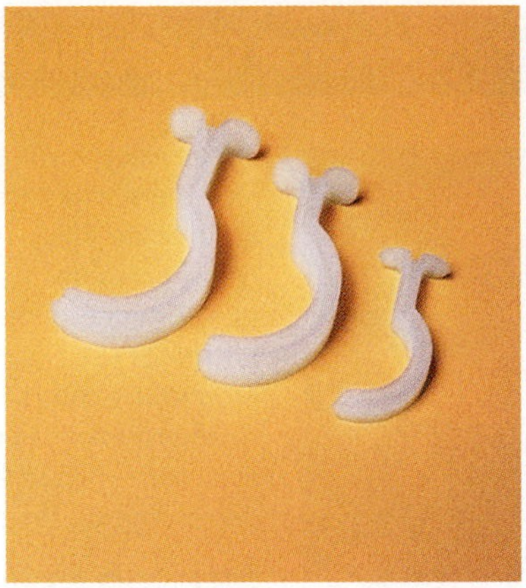

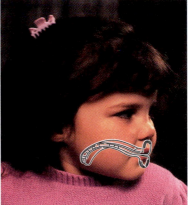

Figure 11-9 *Oropharyngeal airways of various sizes, each with flange, bite block, and curved body.*
Source: www.rnceus.com/hemo/cvp.htm

Figure 11-10 *Estimating the size of an oropharyngeal airway.*

EQUIPMENT AND SUPPLIES

- Oropharyngeal airways of different sizes
- Airway suction equipment

PROCEDURE

1. Carefully assess the child during the procedure.

2. Once the airway is in place, maintain the child's head and jaw in a neutral position, neither flexed forward nor hyperextended. Assess the child's respiratory rate and effort.
   RATIONALE: *This position keeps the trachea from being crimped.*

3. If the child regains consciousness, remove the oropharyngeal airway.
   RATIONALE: *The airway will stimulate the gag reflex and vomiting that can increase the risk for aspiration.*

SKILL 11-9 Assisting with Nasopharyngeal Airway Insertion

The nasopharyngeal airway provides a passage for air in situations when the tongue may fall back into the oropharynx and obstruct the airway. It is used for a conscious child with an obstructed airway, or for a child who potentially may lose consciousness and lose an open airway. The airway is made of soft plastic or rubber and comes in various sizes. The airway must be the correct size. The physician usually inserts the airway in a posterior direction.

PREPARATION

1. Verify the identity of the child. Explain the procedure to the child and parents. Explain that the airway should not be touched to prevent it from being dislodged.

2. Select the correct size nasopharyngeal airway. The length of the tube is determined by measuring the distance from the tip of the nose to the tragus of the ear (Figure 11-11). The width must allow for passage through the nares.

3. Lubricate the tip with water-soluble gel.

EQUIPMENT AND SUPPLIES

- Nasopharyngeal airways of different sizes
- Water-soluble lubricant

PROCEDURE

1. Assist the physician to insert the airway by positioning and holding the child's head at midline in a neutral position, neither flexed forward nor hyperextended.

2. Following insertion of the airway, observe for bleeding in the back of the throat. Blood may exacerbate the obstruction and further compromise airway management.
   RATIONALE: *Insertion of the tube may cause trauma to the nasopharyngeal airway passage.*

3. Assess the child's respiratory rate and effort.

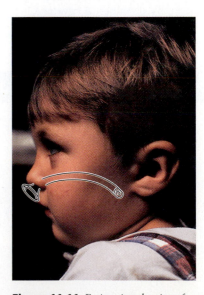

Figure 11-11 *Estimating the size of a nasopharyngeal airway.*

SKILL 11-10 Tracheostomy General Guidelines

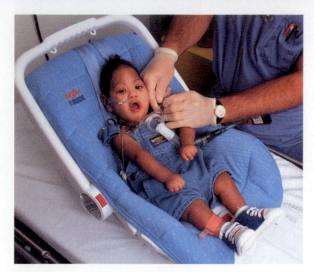

Figure 11-12 *Infant with a tracheostomy collar.*

A tracheostomy is a surgical procedure to make an opening through the neck into the trachea and create an airway. It may be performed by a physician as an acute lifesaving procedure or for management of the child with a chronic disease.

A neonatal or pediatric tracheostomy tube is made of plastic and has an obturator used for insertion only. The tube is held in place with twill tape tied around the child's neck or with Velcro straps. The child usually wears a tracheostomy collar (mist collar) at the stoma site to keep the airway warm and moist (Figure 11-12). The collar may emit either oxygen or room air, depending on the physician's orders.

PREPARATION

1. When a child with a tracheostomy is admitted, plan for close monitoring of the child's respiratory status.

2. Obtain equipment and supplies for any emergency intervention needed.

EQUIPMENT AND SUPPLIES

- Resuscitation bag
- Oxygen
- Sterile suctioning equipment
- Preservative free sterile saline and sterile water
- Water-soluble lubricant
- Tracheostomy tubes—one the size of the child's current tube and one a size smaller, obturator to fit the current tracheostomy tube
- Twill tape or Velcro tracheostomy securing straps

PROCEDURE *Clean Gloves*

1. Observe the child with a tracheostomy carefully for signs of obstruction.

2. Vital signs and respiratory status, including breath sounds, respiratory effort, and airway patency, should be routinely checked. Be alert for changes in heart or respiratory rate, blood pressure, color, or level of consciousness.

3. Watch for condensation in the oxygen tubing and empty it regularly.
   RATIONALE: *Fluid may drip into the tracheostomy tube, causing the child to aspirate if the oxygen tubing is not emptied regularly.*

4. When the child is in a crib, put the tubing through, rather than over, the bars.
   RATIONALE: *This prevents fluid from entering the tracheostomy.*

5. Document findings about the tracheostomy and the child's condition.

CLINICAL TIP

When the child is admitted with a tracheostomy, talk with the parents about the method used for tracheostomy management at home. Develop a nursing care plan for tracheostomy management that integrates home management as well as teaching to enhance home management techniques.

CLINICAL TIP

Always keep a sterile packaged tracheostomy tube taped to the child's bed so that if the tube dislodges, a new one is available for immediate reintubation.

SKILL 11-11 Tracheostomy Care

Tracheostomy care is usually performed two or three times a day. An assistant should always be present while tracheostomy care is being performed. Good stoma care is needed to maintain skin integrity and to help prevent infection.

PREPARATION

1. Verify the identity of the child. Explain or review the procedure with the child and parents.

2. Have an assistant stand on the opposite side of the bed.
   RATIONALE: *For maximum safety two persons should be present for the tracheostomy tube change.*

3. Have prepared tracheostomy tubes, oxygen, resuscitation bag, and suction tray with catheters at the bedside.

4. Prepare new ties for the tracheostomy tube. Cut two pieces of twill tape, about 12 inches each. Fold one end of each piece over lengthwise for approximately 1 to 1 1/2 inches. Cut a

small hole in the folded end. Alternatively use Velcro tracheostomy straps and secure to the tracheostomy.

5. Place a towel roll under the child's neck to hyperextend it.
   RATIONALE: *This provides greater access to the neck, especially in infants and young children who have short necks.*

EQUIPMENT AND SUPPLIES

- Resuscitation bag and oxygen
- Towel roll
- Precut twill tape or Velcro tracheostomy straps
- Cotton-tipped applicators saturated with diluted acetic acid, half-strength hydrogen peroxide, or other preferred cleanser (Lewarski, 2005)
- Cotton-tipped applicators saturated with normal saline
- Gauze pads (some moistened with saline and others dry)
- Scissors
- Sterile curved Kelly clamp
- Tracheal tube cleaning tray with sterile bowls, pipe cleaners, brush, and notched gauze pad
- Sterile hydrogen peroxide, preservative-free sterile normal saline, and sterile water
- Sterile suction tray and catheters
  NOTE: *Equipment is usually available in a prepackaged kit.*

PROCEDURE *Sterile Gloves*

1. Perform hand hygiene.
2. Open sterile suction kit. Pour sterile saline into a sterile bowl and hydrogen peroxide into another bowl.
3. Preoxygenate the child or increase ventilatory support as needed.
4. Don the sterile gloves.
5. Unlock the inner cannula and place it into the bowl containing the hydrogen peroxide. Clean the cannula thoroughly with sterile applicators and rinse in normal saline. Replace the inner cannula and lock it into place.
   RATIONALE: *The inner cannula becomes obstructed with airway secretions and must be cleaned regularly to keep the airway open.*

6. Using cotton-tipped applicators saturated with a neutral pH soap, diluted acetic acid, or another product preferred by the physician, clean under the tracheostomy tube at the stoma site (Fiske, 2004). Start at the stoma and wipe outward with the applicators, making sure no dried or crusted secretions enter the stoma (Figure 11-13). With the tapes still tied, rinse the stoma with saline applicators. Wash the area behind the flanges of the tracheostomy and around the neck with damp gauze, observing for redness, drainage, or skin breakdown. Dry thoroughly.
   RATIONALE: *The airway secretions irritate the skin and cause skin breakdown if not removed regularly.*

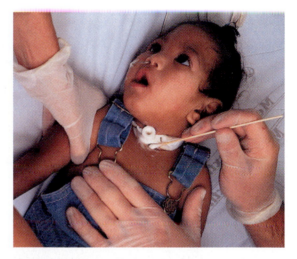

Figure 11-13 *Cleaning the tracheostomy tube.*

7. Place a notched gauze pad under and around the tube.
8. To replace the ties for the tube, have the assistant hold the tube in place. Cut the tapes and remove the old ties from the flange of the tube.
   RATIONALE: *Having an assistant ensures that the tube does not get expelled if the child coughs or moves unexpectedly.*

9. Attach the twill tape to the flange by first threading the end with the slit through the hole. Place the distal end of the twill tape through the slit and pull it securely. Alternatively, attach the Velcro strap to the flange.
10. Have the assistant repeat this step on the opposite side while you hold the tube in place.
11. With the tube held in place, tie the tape or secure the strap. The best fit is achieved when the child's neck is slightly flexed. The tape should be tied tightly enough to prevent dislodgment but should still be loose enough so that you can fit one finger between it and the child's neck.
12. Double- or triple-knot the tape for security. Place the knot at the side of the child's neck.
    RATIONALE: *This prevents skin irritation from the knot when the child is supine.*
13. Document the procedure, the condition of the tracheostomy opening, and how the child tolerated the procedure.

CLINICAL TIP

Remember that the child with an endotracheal tube or tracheostomy tube is unable to talk or cry. Implement other ways of communication. Picture boards with common activities or requests work for younger children. A tablet and pencil can be used by older children with normal motor function.

SKILL 11-12 Endotracheal Tube Care

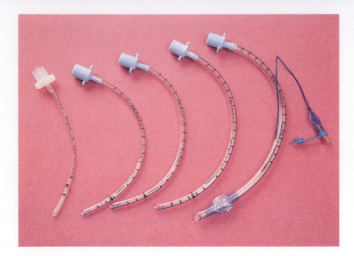

Figure 11-14 *Endotracheal tubes.*

An endotracheal tube is an emergency artificial airway used to maintain and secure an open airway in an unconscious child. Endotracheal (ET) tubes are sterile, disposable, and made of a translucent plastic or other synthetic material. The distal end is tapered and has an opening in the side wall (Murphy's eye). The length of the tube is marked in centimeters to serve as a measurement reference point once it is in place. The tubes come in various sizes, both with and without cuffs (Figure 11-14). The uncuffed tube is recommended for the child younger than 8 or 9 years old, since the airway is narrowest at the cricoid ring, sealing the airway effectively without a cuff. Intubation is usually performed by the physician or paramedic to maintain the child's airway.

PREPARATION

1. Verify the identity of the child and explain the procedure to the parents (the child will be unconscious or less than fully responsive).

2. Select the appropriate size tube for the child. Use a length-based resuscitation tape or formula to select tube size. See Table 11-3. The size of the tube can be approximated by comparing it with the diameter of the child's fingernail on the fifth finger. The formula used for children older than 2 years of age is:

   (16 plus age in years) divided by 4 equals the size of ET tube

3. Place the child in the supine position with the neck hyperextended (unless there is concern of cervical spine injury, in which case the neck is not hyperextended).

TABLE 11-3	Suggested Endotracheal Tube and Suction Catheter Sizes	
Age	**Endotracheal Tube Size (millimeters)**	**Suction Catheter Size (French)**
Premature newborn	2.0–2.5	5
Newborn	3.0–3.5	6–8
6 months	3.5	8
12–18 months	4.0	8
3 years	4.5	8
5 years	5.0	10
6 years	5.5	10
8 years	6.0	10
12 years	6.5	10
16 years	7.0–8.0	12

Source: Adapted from Dieckman, R. and the American Academy of Pediatrics. (2006). Pediatric education for prehospital professionals. (2nd ed.). Sudbury, MA: Jones & Bartlett. www.jbpub.com. Reprinted with permission.

EQUIPMENT AND SUPPLIES

- Endotracheal tubes of different sizes, cuffed and uncuffed
- Pediatric stylet
- Length-based resuscitation tape
- Adhesive tape
- Laryngoscope with curved and straight blades of different sizes
- Water-soluble lubricant
- CO_2 detector
- Resuscitation bag and oxygen source
- Suction catheter and suction source
- Stethoscope

PROCEDURE *Clean Gloves, Gown, Eye Protection*

1. Assist the physician with intubation by positioning and holding the child's head at midline. The tube is held in position until taped securely.
   RATIONALE: *The position of the tube can easily shift with movement of the child's head and neck. Correct placement of the tube in the trachea is critical for survival of the child.*

2. Once the tube has been placed by the physician, auscultate for equal breath sounds, and check for symmetry of chest movement and condensation in the tube. Attach a CO_2 detector to assess tube placement. Auscultate over the abdomen for any bubbling or gurgling sounds to ensure that the tube is not in the esophagus. Listen at the trachea for air leaks.

3. Once correct tube placement is verified, note the centimeter marking at the lip or tooth line and tape the tube in place.
   RATIONALE: *Identifying the level of tube placement provides one method of confirming placement of the tube during future assessments.*

4. Reassess tube placement after the tube is taped.

5. Continuously assess breath sounds, color, heart rate on the monitor, and pulse oximeter readout.
   RATIONALE: *The child with an endotracheal tube needs constant assessment to ensure that the tube does not become dislodged from the trachea.*

6. Initiate assisted ventilation if spontaneous breathing is not present.

7. Document endotracheal tube insertion, procedures for verification of correct placement, centimeter marking at the teeth or lips, tube size, and the patient's response.

Assisted Ventilation

SKILL 11-13 Bag-Valve-Mask (BVM) Ventilation

Resuscitation bags and masks are used to perform assisted ventilation for the child who is unable to breathe adequately on his or her own. This is an emergency procedure, performed until airway control is attained and a ventilator is provided.

PREPARATION

1. Select the appropriate-size mask for the child. The mask should extend from the bridge of the nose to the cleft of the chin (Figure 11-15).
   RATIONALE: *The correct-size mask has a small volume that minimizes dead space and prevents rebreathing of expired carbon dioxide.*

2. Select the appropriate-size resuscitation bag for the child. The pediatric bag should have a volume of 450 to 750 mL. An adult bag (1200 mL) can be used with older children.
   RATIONALE: *Pediatric tidal volume is approximately 8 mL/kg. The bag size should be no smaller than the child's tidal volume.*

3. Connect the oxygen tubing to the resuscitation bag, and to the flow meter. Set the oxygen flow to 15 L/min.

4. If the resuscitation bag has a pop-off valve, block it.
   RATIONALE: *This allows higher inspiratory pressures to be achieved when used to ensure chest rise.*

EQUIPMENT AND SUPPLIES

- Self-inflating resuscitation bag and appropriate-size mask for child
- Oxygen and tubing
- Appropriate-size suction catheters and suction source
- Pulse oximeter
- Oropharyngeal or nasopharyngeal airway

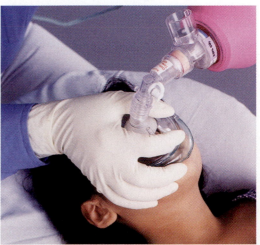

Figure 11-15 *Bag-valve mask. Note the position of the fingers on the mask and jaw to seal the mask to the face.*

PROCEDURE *Clean Gloves*

1. Assess the child's respiratory status, and initiate assisted ventilation when the child is unable to breathe at an adequate rate or depth. Activate the emergency response system in the agency.

2. Open the child's airway with a head tilt–chin lift or jaw thrust maneuver (see Skill 11-18). Use an oropharyngeal or nasopharyngeal airway if airway patency cannot be maintained.

3. Place a towel roll under the infant's or toddler's shoulders to achieve a sniffing position. Avoid hyperextending the neck.
   RATIONALE: *The head of the infant and toddler is large, and lifting the shoulders places the airway in a neutral position.*

4. Apply the mask to the face and get an airtight seal. Pull the child's jaw into the mask rather than pushing the mask into the face. Use an assistant to maintain the seal. The resuscitator bag may also be attached to the child's endotracheal tube.
   RATIONALE: *Failure to achieve a seal will result in a lower oxygen concentration or inadequate volume of air delivered to the lungs.*

5. Begin ventilation by squeezing the bag. Watch for chest rise. Squeeze the bag only until the chest rise is visible, then release.
   RATIONALE: *Using more force than needed to make the chest rise will push air into the stomach and potentially cause the child to vomit, compromising the airway.*

6. With each ventilation, say "squeeze, release, release." The rate of ventilation should be 30/min in infants and 20/min in children.
   RATIONALE: *The child needs a 1:2 inspiratory to expiratory ratio for gas exchange in the alveoli, and this phrase provides a reminder.*

7. Assess the effectiveness of ventilations by observing for bilateral chest rise, auscultating lung sounds, and monitoring pulse oximeter level.

8. Document the procedure and the child's condition.

CLINICAL TIP

Gastric distention can occur with either mouth-to-mouth or resuscitation bag and mask rescue breathing. This distention compromises ventilation by elevating the diaphragm and decreasing lung size. It may also stimulate vomiting. An orogastric tube may be inserted to prevent vomiting.

SKILL 11-14 Ventilator

Ventilators are used for children who need assistance with breathing. These children may have a chronic condition, such as a neuromuscular disease or persistent lung pathology, or they may be acutely ill or injured and need emergency management of ventilation. The ventilator is usually attached to the child's endotracheal tube or tracheostomy tube.

PREPARATION

1. Verify the physician's order.

2. Become familiar with the ventilator, and know the settings ordered by the physician (oxygen concentration, humidity, air temperature, pressure, tidal volume, and inspiratory/expiratory ratio and rate). Identify what the alarms mean, and know how to troubleshoot problems.

3. Verify the identity of the child, and explain the procedure to the child and parents.

EQUIPMENT AND SUPPLIES

- Ventilator complete with tubing setup
- Cardiorespiratory monitor
- Pulse oximeter
- Resuscitation bag and mask, appropriate size for child
- Appropriate-size suction catheters and suction source
- Sterile water for suctioning
- Oxygen source
- Nasogastric tube

PROCEDURE

1. Ensure that the child is attached to a cardiorespiratory monitor and pulse oximeter.

2. Measure arterial blood gases prior to ventilation and within 15 minutes after the child has been placed on the ventilator, and thereafter according to the physician's orders.

3. Assess vital signs every hour, including heart and respiratory rates, blood pressure, temperature, and pulse oximeter reading. Auscultate the lungs in all fields to assess for equal breath sounds. Ensure that the child's respiratory rate is consistent with the ventilator setting.

4. An orogastric or nasogastric tube may be inserted.
   RATIONALE: *This keeps the stomach decompressed to keep the child from vomiting and compromising the airway.*

5. Suction the endotracheal tube or tracheostomy tube as necessary. See Skills 11-23 and 11-24.

6. Protect the endotracheal tube by making sure it is well taped and secure. Support the ventilator tubing to decrease traction on the endotracheal tube by attaching the tubing directly to the bed using a gauze roll and a safety pin.

7. Carefully monitor the child to determine if elbow immobilizers are needed to prevent dislodgment of the endotracheal tube. Acutely ill or injured children may be chemically paralyzed and sedated while on the ventilator. If the child has been given paralytics, watch for signs that further sedation or pain medication may be needed (e.g., a rise in heart rate and blood pressure or tearing suggest distress or pain).

8. Listen and look for air leaks. Make sure that the ventilator is firmly attached to the endotracheal tube or tracheostomy tube.

9. Check the reservoir for humidification at least every 8 hours. Refill or replace water as needed. Watch for condensation in the tubing and empty it regularly.
   RATIONALE: *If fluid is not removed from the tubing, it may drip into the endotracheal tube, causing the child to aspirate.*

10. Tell the child what you are planning to do; for example, "I am going to wash your face" or "I am going to move your arms and legs." The child who is sedated or unresponsive may still be able to hear.

11. Support the family by answering their questions. Encourage them to talk to the child and to bring in audiotapes of favorite music or of family members speaking to the child.

12. Document the child's condition frequently according to agency policy.

Chest Tubes

Chest tubes are inserted into the pleural or mediastinal space to drain fluid, blood, or air so the lung can re-expand. Chest tubes may be placed during surgery, postoperatively, or as an emergency. A chest tube may be attached to suction or be sealed to prevent air from re-entering the pleural space. Chest tubes are inserted by a physician.

SKILL 11-15 Assisting with Placement of Chest Tubes

PREPARATION

1. Verify the identity of the child, and explain the procedure to the child and family as developmentally appropriate.

2. Review the patient's medical record related to the need for chest tube placement.
   RATIONALE: *Knowing the reason the chest tube is placed enables the nurse to respond appropriately if the tube is displaced.*

3. Assess the child's respiratory status to obtain the baseline respiratory rate, respiratory effort, breath sounds, and oxygen saturation level. Breath sounds may be diminished over an area of pneumothorax, hemothorax, or pleural effusion.

4. Assess the patient's pain control. Prepare and administer pain medication as prescribed. Local anesthetic may also be used.

5. Prepare the chest tube drainage collection system by filling the water-seal chamber to the level specified by the manufacturer. The suction-control chamber is then filled with sterile water (to a level of 20 cm of water or as specified by the physician).

EQUIPMENT

- Chest tube drainage system
- Sterile water
- Continuous suction regulator
- Marking pen
- Chest tube insertion tray and supplies
- Chlorhexidine, povidone-iodine solution, or other preferred skin preparation
- Drainage catheter (size ordered, 10–24 French)
- Suture 3.0 silk/ethilon
- Dressing preferred by physician (occlusive, nonocclusive, or transparent)
- Sterile gloves
- Sterile connector
- Local anesthetic and syringe
- Banding gum and ties
- Occlusive tape
- Sleeved Kelly clamps (two for each chest tube)
- Adhesive tape
- Safety pins

PROCEDURE *Sterile Gloves, Gown, Eye Protection*

1. Attach the child to a cardiac monitor and pulse oximeter to monitor vital signs during the procedure.
2. Set up the chest tube insertion tray using sterile technique.
3. Position and hold the child on the unaffected side.
4. Monitor the child's vital signs and respiratory status, and compare to baseline during the local anesthetic administration and chest tube insertion.
5. After the chest tube is inserted, maintain sterility while connecting the chest tube to the water-sealed drainage system or suction. Adjust suction to maintain a gentle bubbling in the chamber.
6. Apply an occlusive dressing over the chest tube insertion site.
   RATIONALE: *Occlusive tape and dressing help prevent entry of air into the chest cavity.*
7. Band or secure all tubing connection sites.
8. Reposition the patient. Obtain and assist with the radiograph, if ordered, to clarify placement and effectiveness of the chest tube.
9. Secure the chest tube to the bed with adhesive tape tabs. Keep a bottle of sterile water or normal saline and sleeved Kelly clamps (two per chest tube) at the bedside at all times. Keep Kelly clamps with the child at all times.
   RATIONALE: *Securing the chest tube drainage system reduces tension on the tubing and potential disconnection. In case of dislodgment, clamp the chest tube with a Kelly clamp or place the end of the tube in the sterile solution. This prevents air from entering the pleural space through the chest tube.*
10. Document the procedure, time, amount and color of drainage, and how the child tolerated the procedure.

SKILL 11-16 Care of the Chest Tube

PREPARATION

1. Verify the identity of the child.
2. Assess the child and family's knowledge related to the need for a chest tube. Explain care of the chest tube to the child and family.
3. Assess the client's respiratory status to include respiratory rate, effort, breath sounds, and oxygen saturation level. Breath sounds over the chest tube site may be diminished.
4. Assess the child's pain control. Children may report pain at the insertion site.

EQUIPMENT AND SUPPLIES

- Gloves
- Dressing supplies
- Bottle of sterile water or normal saline
- Sleeved Kelly clamps
- New drainage system (if being replaced)

PROCEDURE FOR CHEST TUBE CARE *Clean Gloves*

1. Perform hand hygiene and apply gloves.
2. Assess the chest tube insertion site. Inspect the dressing around the chest tube insertion site to make sure it is occlusive.
   RATIONALE: *If it is not occlusive, air can leak into the pleural space.*
3. Change chest tube dressings according to hospital policy. Document the amount of drainage and notify the physician if extensive. Palpate the area around the insertion site for crepitus and document its presence and the size of the affected area. Notify the physician if crepitus is present when previously absent or the size of the area affected increases.
   RATIONALE: *Crepitus may indicate subcutaneous emphysema and may cause discomfort to the child.*
4. Check all connections and ensure that they are taped or banded securely.
5. Check drainage tubing to ensure that it is open and straight. The drainage collection device must be positioned below the chest insertion site.
   RATIONALE: *Kinks or loops can prevent the tube from draining properly. The drainage can flow by gravity when the drainage collection device is lower than the insertion site. It also prevents backflow of drainage to the child's chest.*
6. For safety, a bottle of sterile water or normal saline should be at the bedside at all times, and sleeved Kelly clamps (two per chest tube) should be with the child at all times.
   RATIONALE: *If the chest tube is dislodged, the tubing becomes disconnected, or the seal in the collection system is broken, clamp the chest tube with a Kelly clamp or place the end of the tube in the bottle of sterile solution. This reduces the amount of air from entering the pleural space through the chest tube.*
7. If the chest tube is connected to suction, assess the amount of suction set against the amount of suction ordered. Bubbling in the suction chamber should be gentle rather than continuous. Continuous bubbling may indicate an air leak in the system.
8. If there is a water seal chamber: Check for the expected water movement called *tidalling*, the rise and fall of the water according to the child's respirations.
9. Document the type and amount of output hourly or the frequency ordered. Use a marking pen or tape to mark the fluid level, date, and time on the collection container for the running total. The drainage system is never emptied. Drainage systems are large enough to hold drainage from several days. When full, the system is replaced with a new one.
   RATIONALE: *The system would lose its negative pressure if it were opened.*

PROCEDURE FOR CHANGING THE COLLECTION SYSTEM *Clean Gloves*

1. Prepare the new drainage system as described in Skill 11-15.
2. Remove the tape and bands from the chest tube to the old drainage collection system.
3. Direct the child to blow out and then hold his or her breath. Then clamp the chest tube with a sleeved Kelly clamp about 3.5 to 6 cm (1.5 to 2.5 in) from the insertion site.
   RATIONALE: *The clamp prevents air from entering the pleural space through the tube.*
4. Apply gloves.
5. Disconnect the tubing from the old drainage collection device and attach to the new device while keeping the end of the chest tube sterile.
6. Remove the Kelly clamp and tell the child to breathe.
7. Assess the new system for the amount of suction, continuous bubbling (may indicate an air leak), or the presence of tidalling.
8. Band or tape all connection sites, ensuring that the tubing is straight. Secure the tubing to reduce tension on the chest tube insertion site.
9. Assess the child's respiratory status.
10. Document the procedure, time, total drainage and character, and how the child tolerated the procedure.

SKILL 11-17 Assisting with Chest Tube Removal

PREPARATION

1. Verify the identity of the child. Assess patient and family knowledge related to removal of the chest tube. Explain the procedure to the child and family.

2. The chest tube may be clamped for several hours prior to removal to evaluate the child's response.
   RATIONALE: *Clamping the chest tube provides information about how well the child will tolerate having no chest tube.*

3. Assess the patient's baseline respiratory status, including the respiratory rate, effort, breath sounds, and oxygen saturation level.

4. Assess the patient's pain level and administer pain medication 10 to 15 minutes before the procedure.
   RATIONALE: *Many children report pain upon removal of a chest tube.*

5. Prepare the sterile dressing to be placed over the insertion site.

EQUIPMENT

- Sterile gloves
- Suture removal kit or tweezers and scissors
- Antibacterial or occlusive dressing as preferred by physician
- Occlusive tape

PROCEDURE *Sterile Gloves*

1. Position the child and have an assistant hold the child if necessary.

2. Assist with removal of the dressing and provide reassurance to the child as the dressing is removed.

3. The chest tube may be clamped 3.5 to 6 cm (1.5 to 2.5 in) from the insertion site prior to removal, if not already clamped.

4. As the suture is cut, ask the child to take a breath, blow out, and then hold his or her breath. The chest tube is removed on expiration. If the child is on a ventilator, the chest tube is removed during inspiration.
   RATIONALE: *The diaphragm creates negative pressure in the thoracic cavity on inspiration which would permit air to enter through the chest tube insertion site. A ventilator creates positive pressure in the thoracic cavity during inspiration.*

5. Using sterile gloves, immediately cover the chest tube insertion site with the preferred dressing (occlusive or nonocclusive with antibacterial ointment) and use occlusive tape. Tell the child to begin breathing.

6. Reposition the child and assess breath sounds, respiratory effort, and oxygen saturation level to detect any respiratory distress. Assess pain.

7. Document the procedure, time, child's respiratory status, and how the patient tolerated the removal of chest tube procedure. Document total chest tube output.

8. Assist with the radiograph as ordered following chest tube removal.

Cardiopulmonary Resuscitation

Cardiopulmonary resuscitation (CPR) is basic life support using techniques to maintain airway, breathing, and circulation (the ABCs). CPR guidelines have been revised for children, defined as infants and children up to 14 years of age or the onset of puberty (American Heart Association, 2005). Healthcare professionals should be skilled in both one- and two-person CPR.

SKILL 11-18 Performing Cardiopulmonary Resuscitation

PREPARATION

1. Become certified in basic life support and maintain certification.

2. Assess the child for unresponsiveness, lack of breathing, and no heart rate. Look, listen, and feel for breathing for about 5 to 10 seconds. Check for the rise and fall of the chest and abdomen, and listen and feel for the flow of expelled air at the mouth (Figure 11-16A).
   - Infant: Determine unresponsiveness by gently tapping on the abdomen or soles of the feet. Use the brachial artery to assess for a pulse (Figure 11-16B).
   - Child: Determine unresponsiveness by stimulating the child. Boldly ask, "Are you all right?" Use the carotid artery to assess for a pulse (Figure 11-16C).

3. When to call for help, if none is immediately available:
   - For any child or adolescent with sudden witnessed collapse out-of-hospital, phone for help and send someone to get the automatic external defibrillator (AED) if available.
   - For an unresponsive infant or child with a likely hypoxic arrest (e.g., drowning, injury, drug overdose), initiate CPR for approximately 2 minutes before phoning for help.

EQUIPMENT AND SUPPLIES

- Resuscitation bag and mask
- Mouth-to-barrier device (may be used)

PROCEDURE *Clean Gloves*

Nonbreathing Infant or Child with a Pulse Greater than 60 Beats a Minute

1. If the infant or child is not breathing, give two rescue breaths, about 1 second each, making the chest visibly rise. Seal your lips or mouth-to-barrier device around the child's mouth or around the infant's mouth and nose (Figure 11-17).

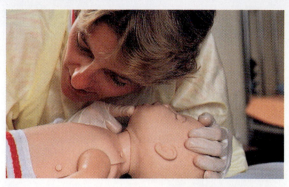

A

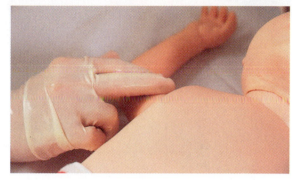

B

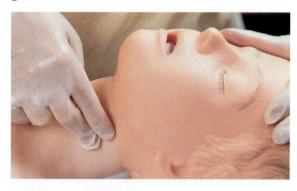

C

Figure 11-16 *A, Assessing breathing. B, Checking for the brachial pulse. C, Checking for the carotid pulse.*

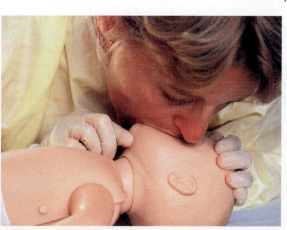

A

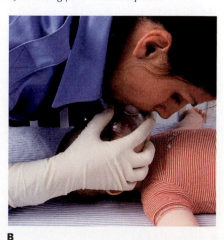

B

Figure 11-17 *A, Mouth-to-mouth-and-nose resuscitation. B, Mouth-to-mouth resuscitation using a barrier device.*

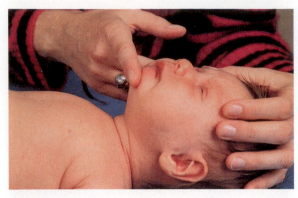

A

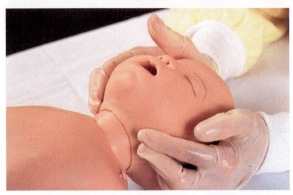

B

Figure 11-18 *A, Head tilt–chin lift maneuver. B, Jaw thrust maneuver.*

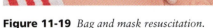

Figure 11-19 *Bag and mask resuscitation.*

- Position the child on the back while supporting the head and neck. Open the airway by performing a chin lift—tilt the head back and lift the chin up and out (Figure 11-18A). A second rescuer should stabilize and maintain the child's head position.
- An alternative procedure for opening the airway on a child suspected of having a cervical spine injury is a jaw thrust—from a position behind the infant's head, the rescuer places two or three fingers under each side of the jaw at its angle and lifts the jaw upward and outward (Figure 11-18B).

2. If the chest does not rise with the first breath, check and adjust the child's position with the chin lift or jaw thrust, and give two effective rescue breaths. If the chest still does not rise, perform the procedure for choking on page 126.

   RATIONALE: *The child could have an airway obstruction.*

3. If the child has a pulse but is not breathing, continue rescue breathing at a rate of 12 to 20 breaths a minute for an infant or child, or 10 to 12 breaths a minute for adolescents and adults. Each breath should cause visible chest rise (American Heart Association, 2005). Recheck the pulse every 2 minutes.

4. Convert to a resuscitation bag and mask hooked up to 100% oxygen as soon as possible (Figure 11-19). Ensure that the mask is the correct size, extending from the bridge of the nose to the cleft of the chin, but not covering the eyes. Continue rescue breathing for as long as the child is not breathing. Use only enough force to make the chest rise. Do not hyperventilate.

   RATIONALE: *Pressure on the eyes stimulates a vagal response, and thus a slowed heart rate. This must be avoided because the child is already compromised.*

Infant or Child with a Pulse Less than 60 Beats a Minute

1. Begin chest compressions after two rescue breaths if the heart rate of an infant or child is less than 60 beats a minute with signs of poor systemic perfusion, despite adequate oxygenation and ventilation.

   RATIONALE: *Bradycardia is a sign of impending cardiac arrest. The rescuer should not wait until the child is pulseless before beginning chest compressions.*

2. Position for chest compressions:
   - The position for compressions in children is about the nipple line. For children use the heel of one or two hands (one hand over the other) for compressions (Figure 11-20). For infants under 1 year of age, the finger position for compressions is one finger's width below the nipple line. Avoid pressure on the xiphoid. For infants, use the two thumbs over the lower sternum and encircle hands around the chest for compressions when two persons are present to perform CPR. The thumbs compress the sternum, and the fingers squeeze the thorax.

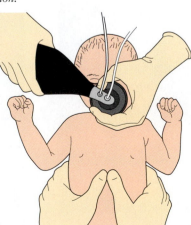

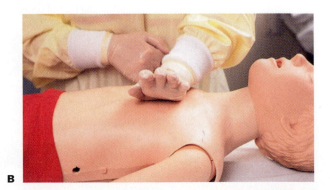

Figure 11-20 *Hand position for chest compressions. A, Infant. B, Child.*   **A**   **B**

3. Perform chest compressions at a rate of 100 per minute, pushing hard to obtain adequate chest compression depth of one third to one half of the chest diameter. Minimize interruptions during compression. Allow the chest to fully recoil after each compression. Compression and recoil time should be about equal (American Heart Association, 2005).

   RATIONALE: *Blood return to the heart is improved if full chest recoil is permitted. Interruptions during compressions reduce blood flow to the brain and the chance for survival.*

4. Single rescuers should use a compression to ventilation ratio of 30 compressions to 2 breaths for all victims regardless of age. When two rescuers are present, the compression to ventilation ratio is 15:2 for infants and children, and 30:2 for adolescents (American Heart Association, 2005).

   - Compressions should be paused for rescue breaths, but interruptions for rescue breaths should be minimized.
   - When an advanced airway such as an endotracheal tube is inserted, compressions are given continuously while the 8 to 10 ventilations are given per minute.

     RATIONALE: *When an advanced airway is in place, ventilations can occur during compressions. A lower than normal respiratory rate is needed to maintain adequate lung perfusion as blood flow to the lungs is lower than normal.*

5. After five cycles (about 2 "CPR minutes"):
   - The single rescuer should interrupt CPR to activate the emergency response system or retrieve an automatic external defibrillator (AED).
   - Multiple rescuers should rotate compressors to reduce rescuer fatigue. Rotation of compressors should occur every 2 minutes, and compressions should be interrupted by no more than 5 seconds.

6. Continue the cycle of compressions and rescue breaths until signs of circulation return or until help arrives with an AED or manual defibrillator.

7. An AED or manual defibrillator should be used as soon as available for the victim with a sudden witnessed collapse. The defibrillator should be used after five cycles of compressions and rescue breaths for all other children over 1 year of age (American Heart Association, 2005).

   RATIONALE: *Sudden collapse in a victim of any age is more likely to be caused by a cardiac condition.*

   - Apply child pads or a child system as directed by the equipment's manual for any child between 1 and 8 years of age (Figure 11-21).
   - Apply adult pads for any child over 8 years of age as directed by the equipment's manual.

8. For the child with ventricular fibrillation, one shock at 2 joules per kg should be immediately followed by five cycles of 15 compressions to 2 breaths. The rhythm is then rechecked. A second shock of 4 joules per kg is given if needed.

9. If the infant or child has a return of both pulse and respirations and is not a trauma victim, place the child in the side-lying position.

   RATIONALE: *This position is used to protect the airway in case of vomiting.*

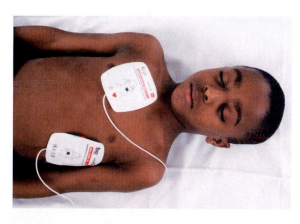

Figure 11-21 *Placement of pads for defibrillation of a child.*

Foreign Body Airway Obstruction

An airway obstruction may be caused by respiratory disorders (e.g., croup or epiglottitis) or a foreign body. Attempts to clear the airway should be made in the following situations: for the witnessed or strongly suspected aspiration of a foreign body or when the airway remains obstructed during attempts to provide rescue breathing.

SKILL 11-19 Removing a Foreign Body Airway Obstruction

PREPARATION

1. When the infant or child is suspected of aspirating, encourage the child to continue crying or coughing and breathing as long as the cough is forceful. Call emergency medical services and try to keep the child calm.

   RATIONALE: *Emergency care should be sought because the infant or child may develop a complete obstruction.*

2. Ask the child, "Are you choking?" If the victim nods, help is needed.

EQUIPMENT AND SUPPLIES

- Mouth-to-mouth and nose barrier device (pocket mask)
- Resuscitation bag and mask

PROCEDURE *Clean Gloves, Mouth-to-Mouth and Nose Barrier Device*

Infant

1. If the cough becomes ineffective and soundless, if increased respiratory difficulty or stridor is noted, or if the infant stops breathing, attempt to remove the obstruction. Use the chin lift position to open the airway.

2. Try to ventilate either by mouth-to-mouth and nose rescue breaths or with a resuscitation bag and mask (refer to Skill 11-18 for rescue breathing and Skill 11-13 for bag-valve-mask ventilation). If the airway is obstructed, reposition the infant's head and attempt to ventilate again.

3. Position the infant face down on your arm supporting the head.

4. Perform five back slaps with the heel of the hand between the infant's shoulder blades (Figure 11-22A).

5. Position the infant face up on your forearm. Place the fingers in the same position used for CPR (Figure 11-22B). Give five chest thrusts near the center of the breastbone.

6. Place your index finger on the bony prominence of the infant's chin and your thumb in the mouth on the tongue. Pull up and out to open the mouth. Look in the infant's mouth for the foreign body and remove it if seen. Do not perform a blind sweep.

   RATIONALE: *A blind sweep may actually push an obstruction deeper into the trachea.*

7. If no object is found, try to ventilate the infant again. If the obstruction is still present, reposition the infant's head and attempt to ventilate once again.

8. If the obstruction remains, begin another series of back blows and chest thrusts. Look in the mouth, try to ventilate, reposition the head, and attempt to ventilate again. Continue with this pattern until the airway is clear.

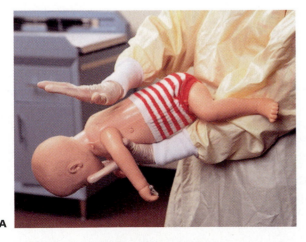
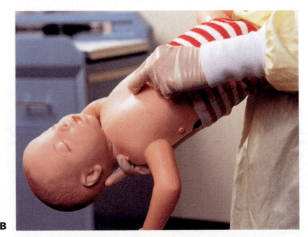

A   B

Figure 11-22 *A, Back slaps. B, Chest thrusts.*

9. If the infant becomes unresponsive, begin CPR as described in Skill 11-18. Every time the rescuer opens the airway to deliver rescue breaths, look in the mouth and remove any object seen. Blind finger sweeps should not be performed (American Heart Association, 2005).

10. Once the airway is clear, give two slow full breaths. Check for a pulse. At this point, provide whatever basic life support (BLS) maneuvers are necessary.

PROCEDURE *Clean Gloves*

Child

1. Perform abdominal thrusts (Heimlich maneuver) on the child in either a sitting or standing position (Figure 11-23).

2. Stand behind the child, with your arms under the child's axilla and around the chest. Place the thumb of one fist against the abdomen in the midline, below the xiphoid and above the navel. Grasp your fist with your other hand.
   RATIONALE: *The xiphoid is avoided to prevent injury to underlying organs.*

3. Deliver up to five quick upward thrusts. Each thrust should be a distinct effort to remove the obstruction.

4. The series of five thrusts should be repeated until the obstruction is cleared or the child becomes unconscious.

5. If the child becomes unconscious, move the child to the floor and begin CPR as described in Skill 11-18. Every time the rescuer opens the airway to deliver rescue breaths, look in the mouth and remove any object seen. Blind finger sweeps should not be performed (American Heart Association, 2005).
   RATIONALE: *Chest compressions during CPR increase the thoracic pressure as high or higher than abdominal thrusts.*

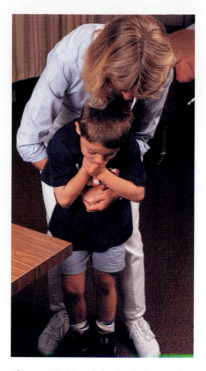

Figure 11-23 *Abdominal thrusts (Heimlich maneuver).*

Suctioning

Suctioning of the airway is needed when excess secretions are present or when a decreased level of consciousness interferes with the child's ability to clear normal secretions. Suctioning of the nose, mouth, tracheostomy tube, or endotracheal tube may all be performed. The size of the suction catheter depends on the size, age, and weight of the child or on the tube requiring suctioning.

Nasal/Oral Suctioning

A bulb syringe is used to remove secretions from an infant's nose or mouth. A tonsil tip or Yankauer catheter may be used for oral suctioning in children when copious, thick secretions or emesis need to be removed.

SKILL 11-20 Performing Nasal/Oral Suctioning

PREPARATION

1. Verify the identity of the child. Explain the procedure to the child and parents.

2. Assess the child's respiratory status, including breath sounds, respiratory effort, and airway patency. Observe for excess secretions that the child is unable to manage by swallowing.

3. An assistant may be needed to gently position and hold the infant or child with the head in midline, and to keep the child's hands out of the way.

4. Turn on and set the wall suction to the pressure level ordered by the physician or suggested in the facility's procedure manual.

EQUIPMENT AND SUPPLIES

- Bulb syringe
- Normal saline nose drops
- Yankauer or tonsil tip suction catheter
- Normal saline solution

PROCEDURE *Clean Gloves*

Bulb Syringe

1. Place saline nose drops in the naris.
   RATIONALE: *The nose drops loosen dried secretions.*

2. Deflate the bulb. Insert the tip of the bulb syringe into the infant's naris (Figure 11-24A).
   RATIONALE: *Deflating the bulb first prevents pushing the secretions back into the nasopharynx.*

3. Release the bulb and remove the syringe from the naris (Figure 11-24B). Expel the secretions into the proper receptacle.

4. Assess the child's ability to breathe easily. Repeat the suctioning as necessary.

5. Document the procedure, character of secretions, and infant's response.

PROCEDURE *Clean Gloves*

Yankauer

1. Insert the catheter tip into the mouth and turn on the suction.

2. Suction to remove secretions from the mouth and pharynx. Avoid causing a gag reflex.
   RATIONALE: *The gag reflex may stimulate vomiting and compromise the airway.*

3. Rinse the catheter with normal saline.

4. Assess the child's respiratory status. Repeat suctioning if needed.

5. Document the procedures, character of secretions, and response of the child.

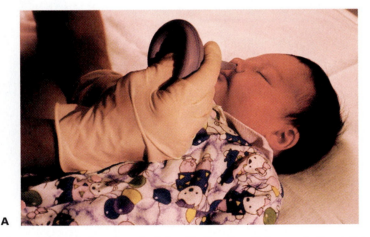
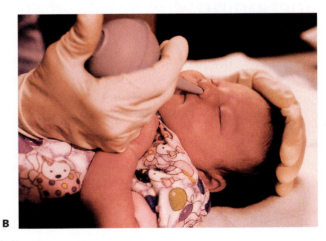

A   B

Figure 11-24 *A, Insertion of a deflated bulb syringe. B, Removal of a reinflated bulb syringe.*

SKILL 11-21 Suctioning a Conscious (Awake and Alert) Child

A catheter is used to remove secretions from an older child's mouth or nose, a tracheostomy tube, or an endotracheal tube. The child with a decreased level of consciousness will likely require deep suctioning to remove secretions (see Skill 11-22).

PREPARATION

1. Verify the identity of the child, and explain the procedure to the child and parents.

2. Have an assistant help you maintain the child's head in the midline position and hold the hands out of the way, as needed. Raise the head of the bed to 30 to 45 degrees.

3. Turn on and set the wall suction to the pressure level ordered by the physician or suggested in the facility's procedure manual.

4. Attach the proximal end of the catheter to the wall suction connecting tubing, making sure to keep the distal end sterile.

EQUIPMENT AND SUPPLIES

- Appropriate-size suction catheter
- Sterile container with preservative-free sterile normal saline
- Suction kit and suction source
- Water-soluble lubricant

PROCEDURE *Sterile Gloves*

1. Keep your dominant hand sterile and your nondominant hand clean for the procedure.

2. With your dominant hand, insert the suction catheter into the child's naris and suction for no more than 5 to 10 seconds, while gently rotating the catheter. (The depth of insertion depends on the size of the child.)

   NOTE: *The mouth may also be suctioned for secretions, but care needs to be taken to avoid stimulating the gag reflex.*

   RATIONALE: *Suctioning longer than 10 seconds causes vagal stimulation and bradycardia.*

3. Remove and irrigate the catheter with sterile normal saline.

4. Assess the child's respiratory status and repeat as necessary.

5. Document the procedure, the character of secretions, and how the child tolerated the procedure.

SKILL 11-22 Suctioning a Child with a Decreased Level of Consciousness

The child with a decreased level of consciousness is unable to get the secretions higher up into the airway. Therefore, deeper suction is often needed to clear the airway.

PREPARATION

An assistant may be needed to keep the child's head in the midline position.

1. Verify the identity of the child, and explain the procedure to the child and parents.

2. Raise the head of the bed to 30 to 45 degrees.

3. Turn on and set the wall suction to the pressure level ordered by the physician or suggested in the facility's procedure manual.

4. Attach the proximal end of the catheter to the wall suction connecting tubing, making sure to keep the distal end sterile.

EQUIPMENT AND SUPPLIES

- Appropriate-size suction catheter (see Table 11-3 on page 116).
- Suction source
- Sterile container with sterile normal saline
- Resuscitation bag and mask
- Oxygen source, tubing, and mask or cannula

PROCEDURE *Sterile Gloves*

1. Place an oxygen mask or cannula on the child's face.

   RATIONALE: *Because suctioning potentially causes hypoxia, oxygenate the child prior to suctioning.*

2. If possible, encourage the child to cough to make the secretions pool in the hypopharynx.

   RATIONALE: *This may prevent the need for deep suctioning.*

3. Keep your dominant hand sterile and your nondominant hand clean for the procedure. Use only the dominant hand to manipulate the catheter.

4. Remove the protective sheath from the catheter, and test the suction by placing it in a cup of sterile saline.

5. Remove the child's oxygen mask or cannula.

6. For nasal/oral suctioning, use your dominant hand to insert the catheter into the child's naris or mouth without occluding the suction port.
   RATIONALE: *This decreases the time of suctioning and reduces the risk for hypoxia.*

7. Slowly advance the catheter only into the hypopharynx. Occlude the suction port and rotate the catheter, applying intermittent suction for 5 to 10 seconds.

8. Remove the catheter and clear the tubing with sterile saline. Repeat as necessary.

9. For deep suctioning, use your dominant hand to insert the catheter (without occluding the suction port) beyond the hypopharynx and into the trachea (the length advanced is determined by the size of the child).

10. When the catheter is in place, gently rotate it while suctioning intermittently. To prevent hypoxia, do not suction for more than 5 to 10 seconds.
    RATIONALE: *Rotating the catheter ensures that the catheter eye has the greatest access to secretions.*

11. Remove the catheter and clear the tubing with sterile saline. Repeat as necessary.

12. Allow the child to breathe normally, and give supplemental oxygen between suctionings.
    RATIONALE: *Because of the risk for hypoxia and bradycardia, give oxygen to improve oxygen status.*

13. Document the procedure, the character of secretions, and the child's response and vital signs.

> **CLINICAL TIP**
>
> Obtain baseline vital signs before and after the procedure. When suctioning, watch for a decrease in pulse rate, an increase or decrease in respiratory rate, or a change in color. Bradycardia may be a sign of vagal stimulation. If any of these signs occur, stop immediately and give the child oxygen using blow-by, a face mask, or mask on the resuscitation bag with attached oxygen source.

SKILL 11-23 Tracheostomy Tube Suctioning

A tracheostomy is an opening through the neck directly into the trachea. It is used to provide adequate ventilation when the child is unable to breathe effectively alone. This is a surgical opening and must be treated carefully to maintain patency, ensure freedom from infection, and promote adequate oxygenation. Suctioning is needed when the infant or child is unable to cough up secretions or has increasing respiratory distress, noisy respirations, color change, tachycardia, or tachypnea (Fiske, 2004).

PREPARATION

1. Verify the identity of the child. Explain the procedure to the child and parents.

2. An assistant or parent may be needed to position and hold the child and to keep hands out of the way.

3. Place the head of the bed at a 30-degree angle.

4. Turn on and set the wall suction to the pressure level ordered by the physician or suggested in the agency's procedure manual.

5. Turn on the oxygen source attached to the resuscitation bag to inflate the reservoir bag so it is ready to use.

6. Attach the proximal end of the catheter to the wall suction connecting tubing, making sure to keep the distal end sterile.

> **CLINICAL TIP**
>
> To determine the appropriate-size suction catheter for a tracheostomy tube, the following formula can be used:
>
> Tracheostomy tube inner diameter × 2 = Suction catheter size
>
> If the calculated size falls between two suction catheter sizes (e.g., 7), select the smaller size catheter (e.g., size 6 rather than the size 8) (Adirim, Smith, & Singh, 2006).

EQUIPMENT AND SUPPLIES

- Additional prepared tracheostomy tubes (see Skill 11-11 for tracheostomy care)
- Resuscitation bag with attached oxygen source
- Appropriate-size suction catheter (see Table 11-3, page 116)
- Suction source
- Sterile container with preservative-free sterile normal saline

PROCEDURE *Sterile Gloves*

1. Keep your dominant hand sterile and your nondominant hand clean for the procedure. Use only the dominant hand to manipulate the catheter. With your dominant hand, remove the catheter from the paper sheath, keeping it sterile.

2. Place the distal end of the catheter in a cup of sterile saline to test the suction.

3. With your nondominant hand, remove the humidity source from the child's tracheostomy tube.

4. Oxygenate the child before suctioning, using a resuscitation bag in your nondominant hand. Give several breaths and remove the resuscitation bag.

5. Using your dominant hand, place the suction catheter into the tube, making sure no suction is being applied at this time. Advance the catheter no farther than 0.5 cm below the edge of the tracheostomy tube.
   RATIONALE: *The tracheostomy tube is already fairly far into the trachea. Going deeper may stimulate a vagal response.*

6. Once the catheter is in place, intermittently occlude the suction port and rotate the catheter to maximize contact between the tube and the side holes of the catheter (Figure 11-25). To prevent the child from becoming hypoxic, do not suction for longer than 5 seconds.

7. Remove the catheter and irrigate it in a cup of sterile saline.

8. Repeat as necessary, oxygenating between suctionings.

9. Alternatively, two people can do the procedure with one applying the resuscitation bag and the other performing suction.

10. Document the procedure, the character of secretions cleared, how the child tolerated the procedure, and vital signs.

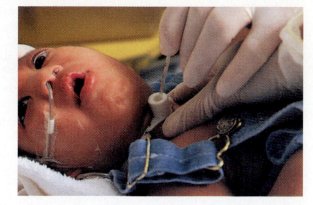

Figure 11-25 *Tracheostomy tube suctioning.*

SKILL 11-24 Endotracheal (ET) Tube Suctioning

The child with an ET tube is often sedated, so deep suctioning may be required to clear secretions that could obstruct the endotracheal tube. It must be performed with great care to keep the tube from being dislodged. Hold the tube firmly in place whenever it is being manipulated: while the ventilator is being disconnected, when the resuscitation bag is being attached and removed, during hyperventilation, and during suctioning.

PREPARATION

1. Verify the identity of the child. Explain the procedure to the parents, and to the child if alert.

2. Use an assistant to help stabilize the ET tube during the procedure.

3. Turn on and set the wall suction to the pressure level ordered by the physician or suggested in the facility's procedure manual. Connect the proximal end of the catheter to the wall suction connecting tubing.

4. Turn on the oxygen source attached to the resuscitation bag to inflate the reservoir bag so it is ready for use.

EQUIPMENT AND SUPPLIES

- Appropriate-size suction catheter to fit inside the ET tube (See Table 11-3, page 116)
- Sterile container with sterile preservative-free normal saline
- Resuscitator bag
- Oxygen source and tubing

PROCEDURE *Sterile Gloves*

1. Keep your dominant hand sterile and your nondominant hand clean for the procedure. Use only the dominant hand to manipulate the catheter.

2. With your dominant hand, remove the catheter from the paper sheath, keeping it sterile. Place the distal end of the catheter in a cup of sterile saline to test the suction pressure.

3. If the child is being ventilated, have an assistant disconnect the ventilator and manually ventilate and oxygenate the child before suctioning with the resuscitator bag. Give several breaths and then remove the resuscitation bag.

4. Before inserting the catheter, determine how far the suction catheter can be advanced by making a visual comparison of the catheter and the ET tube length.
   RATIONALE: *The visual comparison between the catheter and ET tube length allows for preplanning of how far to advance the catheter to prevent damage to the airway.*

5. With your dominant hand, place the suction catheter into the ET tube, making sure that no suction is being applied at this time. Advance the catheter no farther than 0.5 cm below the edge of the ET tube.

   RATIONALE: *Advancing the catheter beyond this distance has the potential to cause damage to the airway and lungs.*

6. When the catheter is in place, intermittently cover the suction port and rotate the catheter. To prevent the child from becoming hypoxic, do not suction for longer than 5 to 10 seconds.

7. Remove the catheter and irrigate it in a cup of sterile saline. Repeat as necessary, assessing the child's vital signs and oxygenating the child between suctionings.

8. Document the procedure, the secretions cleared, their color and quality, how the child tolerated the procedure, and vital signs.

Chest Physiotherapy/Postural Drainage

Chest physiotherapy is an airway clearance technique that combines positioning or postural drainage (allowing gravity to help drain secretions into central airways), rhythmic percussion of the chest wall (to help loosen secretions), and coughing and breathing. Chest physiotherapy is used in children who have excessive sputum production or retained bronchial secretions.

These procedures are usually done before the morning meal, and again at bedtime if the child is subject to nighttime mucus retention, plugging of airways, and/or coughing. Chest physiotherapy may be performed more frequently when an infection is present.

Bronchodilators are frequently administered by a handheld nebulizer, intermittent positive pressure breathing (IPPB), or a metered-dose aerosol before drainage is performed.

Two maneuvers can be done to aid in postural drainage: percussion and vibration. Percussion produces chest vibrations that dislodge retained secretions. Vibration is the application of a downward vibrating pressure with the flat part of the palm over the area that is being drained. Some children with cystic fibrosis use a vest airway clearance system (Figure 11-26). The vest provides high-frequency chest wall oscillation that increases airflow velocity to create repetitive cough-like shear forces and decrease the viscosity of secretions. The vest is used in 30-minute sessions (Goodfellow & Jones, 2002).

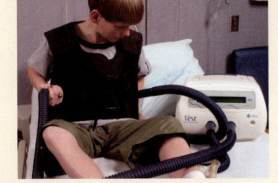

Figure 11-26 *Child with cystic fibrosis using a vest for chest physiotherapy.*

SKILL 11-25 Performing Chest Physiotherapy/Postural Drainage

PREPARATION

1. Verify the identity of the patient, and review the procedure with the child and parents.

2. Ensure that several hours have passed since the child has eaten.

   RATIONALE: *Percussion stimulates coughing spells that can trigger vomiting. Vomiting is less likely if the stomach is empty.*

3. Perform a baseline respiratory assessment. Place the child on a pulse oximeter.

   RATIONALE: *Chest physiotherapy predisposes the child to arterial desaturation. A baseline assessment is performed to contrast with the child's responses during the procedure.*

4. Place the child in the position to permit gravity drainage of secretions.

5. Administer the bronchodilator, if ordered, to relax the airway muscles.

   RATIONALE: *When the airway muscles are relaxed, the airway is more dilated so secretions can drain easily.*

EQUIPMENT AND SUPPLIES

- Commercial percussor, round oxygen mask, baby bottle nipple (for infants)
- Vibrator or vibration vest
- Emesis basin or sputum cup
- Pulse oximeter
- Paper tissues

PROCEDURE *Percussion*

1. If using the hands to percuss the chest, hold the hands cupped with fingers and thumb together. Keep the wrists loose and elbows partially flexed. Strike the chest, alternating the hands. Listen for a hollow sound (see Figure 11-27A and B).

2. Develop a rhythm with the alternate hands, and cover the targeted chest area in a circular pattern for 3 to 5 minutes.

3. Avoid tender areas, the breasts of an adolescent girl, and bony prominences such as the clavicles or vertebrae.

   RATIONALE: *Percussion should be focused over intercostal spaces to have the best effect in loosening secretions. Avoiding tender areas will minimize the child's discomfort.*

4. Have the child change position to drain another area of the lungs and percuss that area for 3 to 5 minutes. Continue this process until all areas of the chest have been percussed.

5. The positions used for each patient are based on the location of mucous obstruction (see Table 11-4). In generalized obstructive lung disease, the lower lobes are drained first, followed by the middle lobes and lingula. The upper lobes are drained last. The various positions used for bronchial drainage in an infant are described in Table 11-5 on page 136.

6. Encourage the child to take a few deep breaths and to cough after percussion in each location. Have the child expectorate sputum into an emesis basin or cup.

   RATIONALE: *The deep breaths increase the velocity of expired air and help to move the secretions toward the trachea where they can be coughed up.*

7. Monitor the child's cardiorespiratory status.

8. Document the procedures, quality of expectorants, and how the child responded to the procedure.

PROCEDURE *Vibration*

1. Position one hand flat on the chest over the involved area and the other hand on top of the first. Alternatively the hands may be placed side by side on the chest. Keep the arms and shoulders straight.

2. Tell the child to take a deep breath, inhaling through the nose and exhaling through the mouth.

   RATIONALE: *Vibration is performed only during exhalation.*

3. Vibrate the area by tensing and relaxing your arms for 10 to 15 seconds. Perform these tensing/relaxing actions for 3 to 5 minutes. Move to another area of the chest and repeat the process (Figure 11-27C).

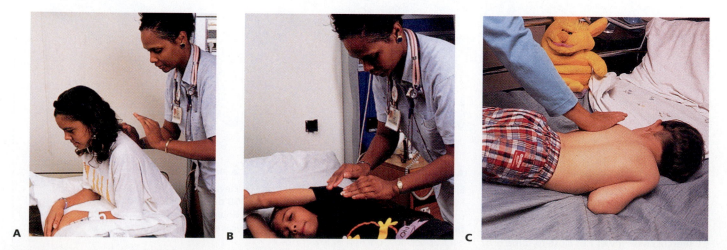

A   B   C

Figure 11-27 *A and B, Postural drainage can be achieved by clapping with a cupped hand on the chest wall over the segment to be drained to create vibrations that are transmitted to the bronchi to dislodge secretions. Various positions are used, depending on the location of the obstruction (see Table 11-4). C, Vibration technique of chest physiotherapy.*

TABLE 11-4   Positions Used for Postural Drainage of the Child

Bronchopulmonary segments

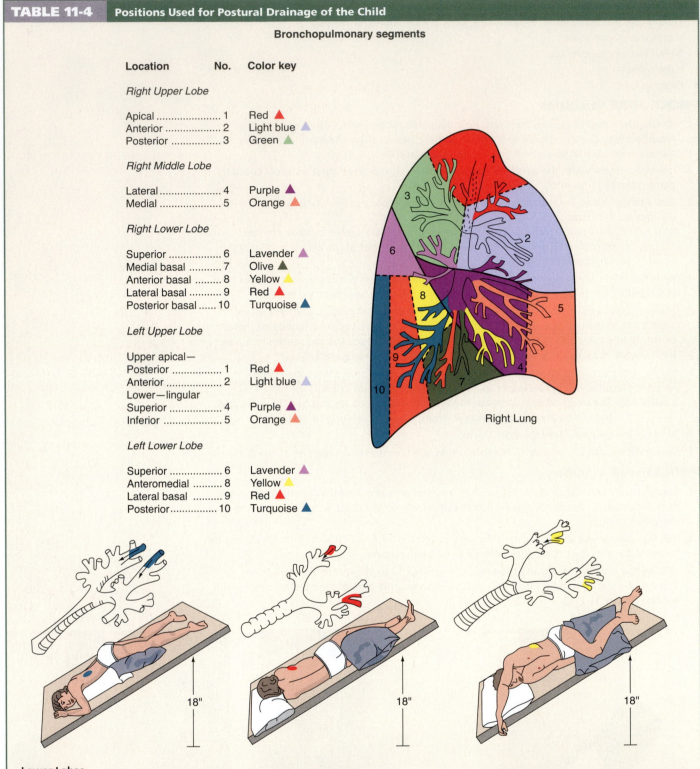

Location	No.	Color key
Right Upper Lobe		
Apical	1	Red ▲
Anterior	2	Light blue ▲
Posterior	3	Green ▲
Right Middle Lobe		
Lateral	4	Purple ▲
Medial	5	Orange ▲
Right Lower Lobe		
Superior	6	Lavender ▲
Medial basal	7	Olive ▲
Anterior basal	8	Yellow ▲
Lateral basal	9	Red ▲
Posterior basal	10	Turquoise ▲
Left Upper Lobe		
Upper apical—		
Posterior	1	Red ▲
Anterior	2	Light blue ▲
Lower—lingular		
Superior	4	Purple ▲
Inferior	5	Orange ▲
Left Lower Lobe		
Superior	6	Lavender ▲
Anteromedial	8	Yellow ▲
Lateral basal	9	Red ▲
Posterior...............	10	Turquoise ▲

Right Lung

Lower Lobes

▲ Posterior Basal Segment (10)

Elevate foot of table or bed 18 in. or 30 degrees. Have child lie prone, head down, with pillow under hips. Upper leg can be flexed over a pillow for support. (Percuss over lower ribs close to spine on each side of chest.)

▲ Lateral Basal Segment (9)

Elevate foot of table or bed 18 in. or 30 degrees. Have child lie prone, then rotate 1/4 turn upward. Upper leg can be flexed over a pillow for support. (Percuss over uppermost portion of lower ribs.)

▲ Anterior Basal Segment (8)

Elevate foot of table or bed 18 in. or 30 degrees. Have child lie on side, head down, pillow under knees. (Percuss over lower ribs just beneath axilla.)

(continued)

TABLE 11-4   Positions Used for Postural Drainage of the Child—*Continued*

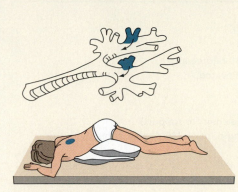

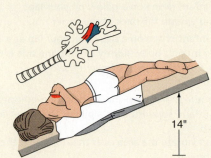

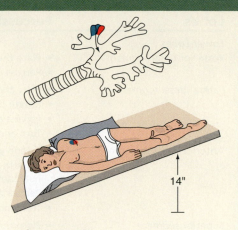

Lower Lobes—cont'd

▲ *Superior Segment (6)*

Place bed or table flat. Have child lie with pillows under hips. (Percuss over middle of back below tip of scapula on either side of spine.)

Right Middle Lobe

▲ *Lateral Segment (4)*

▲ *Medial Segment (5)*

Elevate foot of table or bed 14 in. or about 15 degrees. Have child lie head down on left side and rotate 1/4 turn backward. Pillow may be placed behind child from shoulder to hip. Knees should be flexed. (Percuss over right nipple area.)

Left Upper Lobe

▲ *Lingular Segment—Superior (4)*

▲ *Inferior (4)*

Elevate foot of table or bed 14 in. or about 15 degrees. Have child lie head down on right side and rotate 1/4 turn backward. Pillow may be placed behind child from shoulder to hip. Knees should be flexed. (Percuss over left nipple area.)

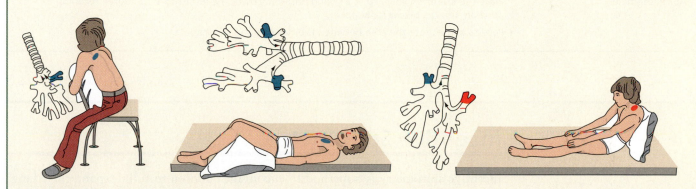

Upper Lobes

▲ *Posterior Segment (3)*

Have child sit up and lean over folded pillow at 30 degree angle. (Percuss over upper back on each side of chest.)

▲ *Anterior Segment (2)*

Place bed or drainage table flat. Have child lie supine with pillow under knees. (Percuss between clavicle and nipple on each side of chest.)

▲ *Apical Segment (1)*

Place bed or drainage table flat. Have child lean back on pillow at 30 degree angle. (Percuss over area between clavicle and top of scapula on each side of chest.)

Data from material provided by Datalizer Slide Charts, Addison, IL.

4. Encourage coughing between vibrations and expectoration of sputum into a cup or emesis basin.

5. Document the procedures, quality of expectorants, and how the child responded to the procedure.

TABLE 11-5	Positions to Facilitate Bronchial Drainage in an Infant
Lobes	**Percussion/Vibration Positions and Locations**
Lower Lobes	
Posterior basal segment	• Place the infant prone on a pillow on your lap. • Percuss and vibrate the back at the lower ribs.
Lateral basal segment	• Place the infant prone on a pillow on your lap at a 30-degree angle. • Rotate the infant's body slightly so that one side is elevated. • Percuss and vibrate over the lower ribs. • Turn and repeat.
Anterior basal segment	• Extend your legs and keep them slightly flexed (use a chair for support). • Place the infant, supported on a pillow, in a side-lying position (30-degree angle) with the head down. • Percuss and vibrate the area over the ribs under the axilla. • Turn and repeat.
Superior segment	• Place the infant prone on a pillow on your lap. • Percuss and vibrate the back.
Upper Lobes	
Lateral and medial segments	• Place the infant on your lap in the prone position. • Rotate the infant slightly so that the right side is elevated. • Percuss and vibrate the anterior chest at the nipple. • Turn the infant and repeat.
Posterior segment	• Place the infant on your lap in a sitting position and leaning forward on a pillow at about a 30-degree angle. • Percuss and vibrate both sides of the upper back.
Anterior segment	• Place the infant supine on your lap. • Percuss and vibrate the area between the clavicle and the midchest at the nipple line.
Apical segment	• Place the infant on your lap in a sitting position. Lower the infant to a 30-degree reclining position, using a pillow for support. • Percuss and vibrate the area between the clavicles and the scapulae.

Incentive Spirometry

Incentive spirometry is a method to encourage children to fully expand their lungs to prevent the pooling of secretions that can occur with inactivity. While it may be ordered by a physician, it can also be a nursing order. Children are often taught incentive spirometry preoperatively so they can effectively use the procedure after surgery.

SKILL 11-26 Using the Incentive Spirometer

PREPARATION

1. Verify the identity of the child. Explain the procedure to the child and parents and why it is important to take deep breaths.
2. Identify the incentive spirometer that matches the child's development.
3. If the child has had thoracic or abdominal surgery, show the child and parent how to splint the surgical site to reduce discomfort.
   RATIONALE: *Giving the child some control and a strategy to manage discomfort will lead to increased compliance with the procedure.*

EQUIPMENT AND SUPPLIES

- Incentive spirometer
- Straw and cotton balls or plastic disk
- Pinwheel

PROCEDURE

1. Assess the child's respiratory status before and after the procedure, including auscultation of the lungs.

2. With the incentive spirometer, have the child take a deep breath, close the lips around the tube, and blow forcefully but steadily into the tube to make the ball rise (see Figure 11-28). The blowing should be maintained a few seconds to keep the ball suspended.

3. Repeat the procedure two to three times several times a day. Encourage the child to make the ball rise higher each time until the highest level is reached. After the highest level is reached, encourage the child to lengthen the time the ball is suspended.

   RATIONALE: *The forced, sustained exhalation helps move secretions to the central airway, making it easier to cough them up.*

4. An alternative method is to have the child use a straw to blow cotton balls or a plastic disk across a table. Make the procedure a game.

   RATIONALE: *Children respond to competitions and will work harder to perform the procedure successfully.*

5. Preschool children may respond to blowing a pinwheel. As the pinwheel's spinning slows, have the child take another deep breath and blow again. Encourage the child to stretch the expiration to make the pinwheel spin longer. When the child is able to blow more forcefully, slowly move the pinwheel farther away.

6. Document the procedure, the child's response, and respiratory status.

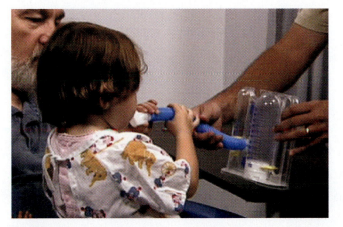

Figure 11-28 *Child using an incentive spirometer.*

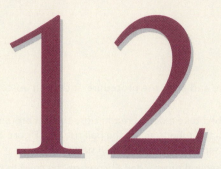

Nutrition

Gastric Tubes

Gastric tubes are used in infants and children to provide a means of alimentation and to decompress or empty the stomach. The size of the nasogastric or orogastric tube is determined by the age, size, and weight of the child.

Orogastric Tubes

Orogastric tubes are used in newborns and young infants who are obligate nose breathers, and in older children who are unconscious, unresponsive, or intubated.

SKILL 12-1 Inserting and Removing an Orogastric Tube

PREPARATION

1. Verify the order and collect supplies.
2. Identify the child and explain the procedure to the child and parent.
3. Assess the child and document findings.

EQUIPMENT AND SUPPLIES

- Appropriate-size orogastric tube
- Suction catheter and equipment
- Water-soluble lubricant
- Stethoscope
- 20-mL syringe to check tube placement

PROCEDURE *Clean Gloves*

Insertion

1. Place the child supine with the head of the bed elevated, unless contraindicated.
2. Use the tube to measure the distance from the mouth to the tragus of the ear and then to the xiphoid process to determine the distance to the stomach. (Alternatively, use a point midway between the xiphoid and the umbilicus.) Mark the tube length for insertion with tape.
3. Have suction at hand. Apply a water-soluble lubricant to the orogastric tube.
   RATIONALE: *If the child vomits, it may be necessary to remove secretions.*
4. Position the child with the neck slightly hyperextended. Open the child's mouth and insert the tube toward the back of the throat. Continue advancing the tube slowly until you reach the mark. Coordinate advancement with swallowing if the child is able to cooperate.
   RATIONALE: *This position facilitates passage of the tube by opening the neck and mouth.*
5. Check the tube for appropriate placement.
   - Aspirate the stomach contents and check the pH of aspirate; a pH of 5 or below generally indicates stomach placement. However, respiratory secretions can have a low pH also so the test is not definitive. Visually evaluate the aspirate as gastric contents are commonly clear or tan.
   - A method of verifying placement after the aspiration test is to use the stethoscope to auscultate over the upper left quadrant of the abdomen while a small amount of air (5 mL or up to 10 mL for an older child) is injected through the tube into the stomach. Air entering the stomach should be heard. Remove air by aspiration after verification.
   - Sometimes a radiograph is used to verify correct placement.
   - Assess the child's respiratory status and color. A change in either or vomiting may indicate that the tube is located in the trachea rather than in the esophagus.
     (Huffman, Jarczyk, O'Brien et al., 2004)
6. Once you are assured that the tube is in place, tape it securely to one side of the child's mouth. Place two pieces of tape in a V pattern around the tube at the lip. If necessary, use a third piece of tape over the other two. Clamp the end of the tube if it is not being used for feeding or suctioning. Repeat assessment of the child.

RATIONALE: *Measures must be taken to maintain the tube in the correct position so that it does not become dislodged.*

7. Document tube placement, length of tube inserted, the child's response, and results of the child assessment.

Removal

1. Verify the identity of the child and explain the procedure to the child and parent.
2. Have suction available.
   RATIONALE: *If the child vomits, it may be necessary to remove secretions.*
3. Instill approximately 10 to 20 mL of air into the tube to remove any secretions.
4. Untape the tube, pinch or fold it to prevent fluid leakage, and gently withdraw it.

Nasogastric Tubes

Nasogastric tubes are used more frequently than orogastric tubes. They are inserted to provide alimentation, to decompress the stomach, or to empty the stomach of its contents in preparation for surgery or lavage.

SKILL 12-2 Inserting and Removing a Nasogastric Tube

PREPARATION

1. Verify the order and collect supplies.
2. Assess the child and document findings.
3. Verify the identity of the child.
4. Tell the preschool-age child what will happen in very simple terms. Give the school-age child and adolescent a rationale for the procedure. Since placement of the tube is uncomfortable, allow the child to express his or her feelings and seek the support of family members.

EQUIPMENT AND SUPPLIES

- Appropriate-size nasogastric tube (see Table 12-1)
- Suction catheter and equipment
- Water-soluble lubricant
- Stethoscope
- 20-mL syringe to check tube placement

PROCEDURE *Clean Gloves*

Insertion

1. Place the child supine, with the head of the bed elevated to the high Fowler position, if possible. Position and hold younger children because they will fight against the insertion of the tube. An assistant can hold the child's body and arms with his or her body, or the child can be put in a modified mummy immobilizer. The child's head will need to be held in the midline position.

TABLE 12-1	Recommended Sizes for Nasogastric Tubes
Age	**Nasogastric Tube Size**
Preterm	5
Newborn and Infant	5–8
1–5 years	8
6–9 years	10
10–12 years	10–12
Adolescent	12 or larger

Source: Reprinted from *Harriet Lane Handbook* (17th ed.) by Robertson, J., & Shilkofski, N. (2005). Copyright 2005, with permission from Elsevier.

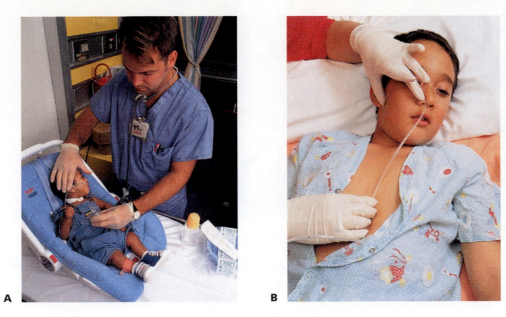

Figure 12-1 *Measuring for nasogastric tube placement in A, an infant, and B, a child. (A similar technique is used in measuring for orogastric tube insertion. See the previous discussion.)*

2. Use the tube to measure the distance from the tip of the nose to the tragus of the ear and then to the xiphoid process to determine the distance to the stomach (Figure 12-1). (Alternatively, use a point midway between the xiphoid and the umbilicus.) Mark the tube length for insertion with tape.

3. Have suction at hand. Apply water-soluble lubricant to the distal end of the nasogastric tube.

4. With the child's neck slightly hyperextended, insert the tube into the child's naris, gently advancing it straight back along the floor of the nasal passages. If resistance is felt at the curve of the nasopharynx, use slight pressure or rotate the tube to continue advancing it.

5. If the child gags when the tube reaches beyond the oropharynx, flex the child's neck. If the child can take fluids by mouth, have him or her sip water through a straw and swallow it to ease the passage of the tube over the glottis. If the child is not allowed anything by mouth, have him or her swallow.

   RATIONALE: *Gagging is most common as the tube passes just beyond the back of the throat. Swallowing can decrease the gag reflex until the tube is advanced slightly beyond this point. This facilitates passage of the tube.*

6. After the gag reflex is suppressed, continue advancing the tube slowly until the marked location on the tube reaches the naris.

7. Check the tube for appropriate placement.
   - Aspirate the stomach contents and check the pH of aspirate; a pH of 5 or below generally indicates stomach placement. However, respiratory secretions can have a low pH also so the test is not definitive. Visually evaluate the aspirate as gastric contents are commonly clear or tan.
   - A method of verifying placement after the aspiration test is to use a stethoscope to auscultate over the upper left quadrant of the abdomen while a small amount of air (5 mL or up to 10 mL for an older child) is injected through the tube into the stomach. Air should be heard entering the stomach. Remove air by aspiration after verification (Figure 12-2).
   - Sometimes a radiograph is used to verify correct placement.
   - Assess the child's respiratory status and color. A change in either or vomiting may indicate that the tube is located in the trachea rather than in the esophagus (Huffman, Jarczyk, O'Brien et al., 2004).

8. Once you are assured that the tube is in place, tape it securely by placing two pieces of tape in a V pattern around the tube and attaching it to the nose or cheek (Figure 12-3). If necessary, use a second piece of tape over the first.

9. Document tube placement, length of tube inserted, the child's response, and results of the child assessment.

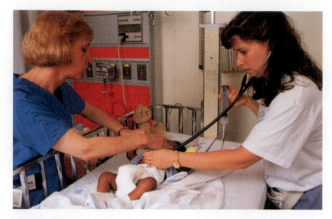

Figure 12-2 *Checking for nasogastric tube placement.*

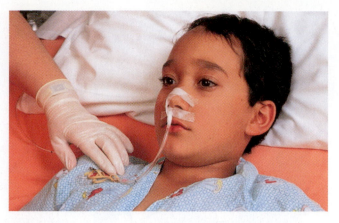

Figure 12-3 *Nasogastric tube taped securely in place.*

Removal

1. Verify the identity of the child and explain the procedure to the parent and child.
2. Have suction available.
3. Place the child in a Fowler position.
4. Instill approximately 10 to 15 mL of air into the tube to remove any secretions.
5. Unfasten the tape, ask the child to hold his or her breath, pinch the tube, and gently pull it out.
6. Document tube removal and the child's response.

Gastrostomy Tubes

Gastrostomy tubes are surgically placed in the stomach and are used primarily for gavage feeding. The tube should remain clamped when it is not being used for feeding or decompression.

Observe the site for skin breakdown. Keep the area clean and dry. Place a clean dry dressing over the site at every shift. A 2 × 2 or 4 × 4 inch gauze pad can be used. A diagonal cut is made halfway into the square and placed around the tube with tape used at the edges to secure it.

Keep the tube as immobile as possible to prevent unintentional removal or displacement. Tube placement can be checked by aspirating a small amount of gastric contents before each feeding.

The gastrostomy feeding button is a flexible silicone device that is often used for children who require long-term enteral feedings.

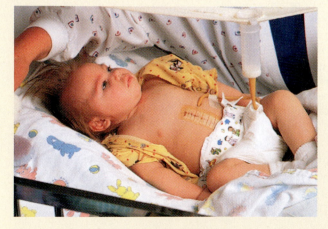

Figure 12-4 *Gavage feeding by gravity.*

Gavage/Tube Feeding

Infants and children require gavage or tube feeding to counteract absorption disorders, to provide supplemental feedings, and to conserve calories for growth. Feedings can be either continuous or bolus. They can be administered by gravity (Figure 12-4) or by pump (Figure 12-5A and B). A pump is preferred because it permits better regulation of the rate and volume of the feeding. While feedings can be administered through orogastric or nasogastric tubes, an indwelling tube is usually surgically placed into the stomach when prolonged feedings will be needed. The tube is often placed by percutaneous endoscopic gastrostomy (and is then called a PEG tube); the tube may be placed in the stomach and be called a gastrostomy (G-tube) or into the jejunum or duodenum and be called a jejunostomy (J-tube). In these cases a balloon or flared tip of the tube is anchored internally into the gastrointestinal system, and a small tube travels outside the body and is anchored on the skin, appearing like a "button."

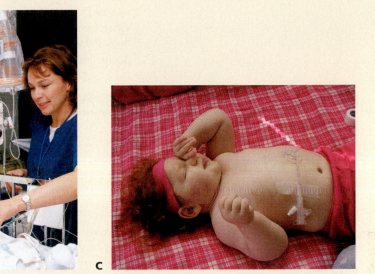

Figure 12-5 *A, Feeding pump. B, The pump helps regulate the rate and volume of feeding. C, A child with feeding tube secured in place.*
© Source anonymous: Used with permission.

SKILL 12-3 Administering a Gavage/Tube Feeding

PREPARATION

1. Verify the identity of the child. Review the feeding procedure with the child and family.

2. If the feeding is to be given by gravity, an IV pole may be used. If the feeding is to be given by pump, gather the necessary bag and tubing. Prime the appropriate tubing, keeping the distal end covered.

   RATIONALE: *The tubing is primed to eliminate air. If air is infused into the gastrointestinal tract, discomfort can occur.*

3. If possible, place the child in a semi-Fowler position. If not, a prone or side-lying position is preferred to the supine position.

   RATIONALE: *These positions decrease the risk of aspiration.*

EQUIPMENT AND SUPPLIES

- Formula at room temperature (to prevent cramping)
- Water for irrigation of the tube
- Stethoscope
- 20-mL syringe to check tube placement

PROCEDURE *Clean Gloves*

1. Check the placement of the tube before each feeding by aspirating the stomach contents or auscultating over the abdomen while a small amount of air (5 mL or 10 mL in older children) is injected through the tube into the stomach. See further methods of assessing for tube placement above.

2. Assess the child's respiratory status and color.

   RATIONALE: *Changes in either may indicate that the nasogastric or orogastric tube is located in the trachea instead of in the esophagus.*

3. Once you are assured that the tube is in place, check gastric residuals and proceed with the steps necessary for the feeding.

Bolus Feeding

1. Aspirate the stomach contents to check the amount of residual. If the residual is less than half of the previous feeding, return the aspirated contents to the stomach. If the residual is greater, notify the physician.

   RATIONALE: *Large residual indicates that the child is not absorbing the feeding. Type or amount may need adjustment.*

2. Attach the primed tubing from either the pump or the gravity set to the gastrostomy tube. Start the flow slowly while checking the patency of the tube. Set the rate and volume according to the physician's orders.

3. When the feeding has been completed, assess the child's condition. Clamp and disconnect the tubing. Flush the tubing with a small amount of water to clean it.

4. When families will carry out tube feedings at home, be sure that they understand the procedure and what to do for any problems (Table 12-2).

5. Document the procedure, gastric residuals, the child's response, and teaching performed.

TABLE 12-2   Home Care Instructions for the Child Requiring Gastrostomy Tube Feedings and Care

Equipment
Prepared, prescribed feeding
Enteral feeding pump
Long-nosed syringe
Clean gloves

Procedure
1. Wash hands.
2. Warm prescribed formula to room temperature.
3. Don gloves and pour formula to run through the feeding bag.
4. Allow formula to run through the tubing to remove air. Close clamp.
5. Attach syringe to the end of the gastrostomy tube. Unclamp the gastrostomy tube.
6. Pull plunger back until resistance is felt. Check amount of formula in syringe. If more than half of the prescribed amount is withdrawn, refer to the section on problem solving in this table. If less than the prescribed amount is withdrawn, push the formula gently back through the syringe.
7. Instill water through the tube.
8. Attach the feeding bag to the gastrostomy tube. Infuse at the prescribed rate.
9. Burp or bubble the infant throughout the feeding.
10. After feeding, flush the gastrostomy tube with water and clamp the tube.
11. Place the infant in the right side-lying position for 1/2–1 hour after feedings if not contraindicated.

Psychosocial Needs
Hold and rock the infant or child during feedings.
Give a pacifier to an infant or a bottle or cup to a child to meet developmental needs.

Medication Administration
Use liquid medication when possible.
Crush only uncoated tablets.
Crush tablets to a fine powder and mix with water or juice.
Flush tubing before and after medication administration.

Stoma Care
Wash the area around the stoma daily with soap and water.
Look for signs of infection, such as redness, swelling, and discharge.
Notify the physician if any signs of infection or leakage are present.

Problem Solving
If the tube comes out, place a dressing over the site and call or visit the care provider or emergency department.
If the tube formula will not flow, make sure the clamp is open. If the clamp is open, try flushing the tube. If this does not resolve the problem, call the number provided at discharge, unless more specific instructions were given at discharge.
If skin breakdown occurs, call for advice before using any creams or ointments, unless specific instructions were given at discharge.
Nurses should provide families with phone numbers to call when complications arise, and Web sites for more information (http://www.kidswithtubes.org).

Source: Table partially compiled by Kay Cowen, RNC, MSN. Data from Borkowski, S. (2005, May). Irritation, redness, and drainage at the site of a pediatric gastrostomy. *The Clinical Advisor,* 90–91; Burd, A., & Burd, R.S. (2003). The who, what, why and how-to guide for gastrostomy tube placement in infants. *Advances in Neonatal Care, 3,* 197–205; Gracey, K., Burd, A., & Burd, R. (2003). Guide for home gastrostomy tube care. *Advances in Neonatal Care, 3,* 206–207; Holmes, S. (2004). Enteral feeding and percutaneous endoscopic gastrostomy. *Nursing Standard, 18* (20), 41–43.

Continuous Feeding

1. The procedure for continuous feeding is very similar to that for bolus feeding. However, the formula should hang no longer than 4 hours.

    RATIONALE: *Microorganisms can grow in warm formula, so it must be changed once left out for several hours.*

2. When the feeding bag is hung, label it with the time and date.

3. Change the feeding set once per shift or every 8 hours.

4. Assess the child's condition and monitor respiratory status during the feeding.

5. Document the procedure and the child's response.

Gastric Suctioning

Both orogastric and nasogastric tubes can be connected to a suctioning device (Figure 12-6) to provide either continuous or intermittent suction.

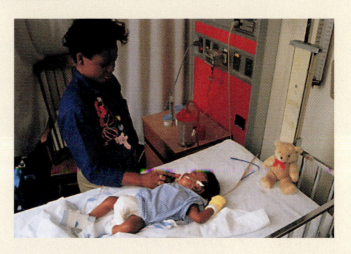

Figure 12-6 *Nasogastric tube attached to a suctioning device.*

SKILL 12-4 Performing Gastric Suctioning

PREPARATION

1. Verify the identity of the child, and explain the procedure to the child and parent.

2. Check the suction equipment.

EQUIPMENT AND SUPPLIES

- Suctioning equipment
- Stethoscope
- 10-mL syringe for air insertion

PROCEDURE *Clean Gloves*

1. Before making the connection, don gloves.

2. Check the tube for proper position by aspirating the stomach contents or auscultating over the abdomen while a small amount of air (5 mL or 10 mL in older children) is injected through the tube into the stomach.

3. Assess the child's respiratory status and color. Changes in either may indicate that the tube is located in the trachea instead of in the esophagus.

4. Attach the suction to the orogastric or nasogastric tube at its distal end. Tape the connection site.

5. Turn the suction to the setting ordered by the physician. Observe the color, amount, and character of the contents suctioned.

6. Document the child's response (vital signs, complaints of abdominal discomfort).

7. Monitor the child's condition frequently, and label the level of the contents collected.

    RATIONALE: *Contents can indicate difficulty absorbing nutrients or suggest problems with digestive processes. In the case of suction following poisoning, contents can indicate the amount of a poisonous substance that has been successfully removed.*

8. Document the procedure and the child's response.

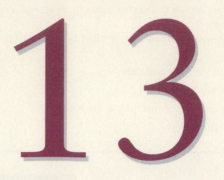

Elimination

CHAPTER OUTLINE

Urinary Catheterization

Urinary catheterization is performed to obtain sterile urine for diagnostic purposes, to measure the amount of urine in the bladder accurately, to empty the bladder, or to relieve bladder distention. In the hospital setting, it is performed as a sterile procedure. For children outside the hospital who need intermittent catheterization, it is done as a clean procedure.

SKILL 13-1 Performing an Indwelling Urinary Catheterization

An indwelling urinary catheterization is performed when urine output needs to be carefully measured, or the bladder needs to be continuously drained.

PREPARATION

1. Check the physician's orders to confirm that indwelling catheterization is planned.
2. Verify the identity of the child. Explain the procedure to the child and parent and why it is necessary.
3. Determine the size of the catheter based on the child's size, age, and weight.

EQUIPMENT AND SUPPLIES

- Urinary catheter—size appropriate for the child's age, and one a size smaller
- Sterile urinary catheterization tray (containing drapes, sterile gloves, antiseptic solution, cotton swabs or balls, forceps, lubricant, and a container for urine)
- Container for soiled cotton balls
- Syringe filled with normal saline
- Tape
- Drainage collection apparatus
- Absorbent pads

> **CLINICAL TIP**
>
> Recommended urinary catheter sizes:
>
> Infant—4–5 French
>
> Toddler and preschooler—6 French
>
> School-age child—6–10 French
>
> Adolescent—8–12 French

PROCEDURE *Sterile Gloves*

1. Have an assistant hold the child in position for the procedure. If the parents wish to stay with the child, have them stand at the child's head and offer distraction and comfort.
2. Place absorbent pads under the child's perineum.
3. Open the tray, maintaining the sterile field. Open the lubricant and squeeze it onto the sterile field. Pour the antiseptic over the cotton swabs or balls.
4. Put on sterile gloves. Lubricate the tip of the catheter and place the distal end in the tray.

Female

5. Clean the perineum. Spread the labia apart with the nondominant hand. Pick up the antiseptic-soaked cotton balls with forceps using the dominant hand. Clean the meatus, using one ball for each wipe, in a front to back direction along each side of the labia minora, then along the sides of the urinary meatus, and finally straight down over the urethral opening. Discard each cotton ball away from the sterile field.
   RATIONALE: *Wiping in the direction from the urinary meatus toward the anus avoids contaminating the urinary meatus with fecal bacteria.*
6. Pick up the lubricated catheter tip with your dominant hand, keeping the distal end in the specimen container.
   RATIONALE: *The dominant hand remains sterile and should be the one to handle the catheter. Placing the distal end in a specimen container prevents contamination of the sterile field when urine flows.*
7. Gently insert the tip into the meatus (approximately 5 to 8 cm [2 to 3 in] in the child) until there is a free flow of urine, and then 2.5 cm (1 in) further (Figure 13-1). If resistance is felt, do not force the catheter. Rotate the catheter gently between your fingers and gently advance. If unsuccessful, try again with another sterile catheter, preferably one size smaller.
   RATIONALE: *A catheter should not be used a second time to prevent potential infection in the child.*

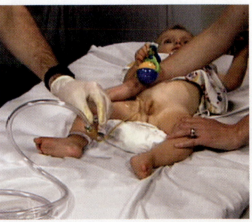

Figure 13-1 *Attaching the catheter to the drainage apparatus, after performing an indwelling urinary catheterization.*

8. When the catheter is in place, collect any needed urine specimen as described in Skill 7-10. Attach the tubing to the drainage apparatus. Tape the tubing to the leg to avoid pulling.

9. Use the syringe to inflate the balloon on the catheter to the recommended amount of normal saline.

10. Make sure the tubing has no kinks. Hang the drainage apparatus on the bed frame below the child.

11. Document the procedure and how the child tolerated it.

CLINICAL TIP

If catheterization is performed for bladder distention, rapid drainage can cause a vasovagal response. Take vital signs before beginning the procedure to establish a baseline. Monitor the child, and clamp the catheter if signs of decreased alertness or lethargy are noted. Once normal assessment findings are reached, slow drainage of urine can resume.

Male

5. Clean the perineum. Retract the foreskin if the child is uncircumcised. With the nondominant hand, hold the penis behind the glans and spread the meatus with your thumb and forefinger.

6. Use the dominant hand to pick up the forceps and antiseptic-soaked cotton balls. Clean the tissue surrounding the meatus using one cotton ball for each wipe in an outward circular motion. Discard each cotton ball away from the sterile field.

7. Pick up the lubricated catheter tip with the dominant hand, and place the distal end in a specimen container. Lift the penis, exerting slight traction until it is perpendicular to the body. Insert the catheter steadily into the meatus until urine begins to flow, and then about 2.5 cm (1 in) further (up to a total of 10 to 12 cm [5 to 6 in] maximum).

   RATIONALE: *The catheter is inserted an extra inch into the bladder to ensure proper placement for drainage when an indwelling catheter is planned.*

8. If resistance to the catheter is felt, have the child blow out to relax the perineal muscles, or rotate the tube between your fingers and gently advance. Do not force the catheter. Another catheter, one size smaller, may be used if relaxation efforts are not successful in advancing the catheter.

9. Once the catheter is in place, lower the penis and collect the urine specimen as described in Skill 7-10. Attach tubing to the drainage apparatus. Tape the tubing to the leg to avoid pulling.

10. Use the syringe to inflate the balloon on the catheter to the recommended amount of normal saline.

11. Make sure the tubing has no kinks. Hang the drainage apparatus on the bed frame below the child.

12. Document the procedure and how the child tolerated it.

SKILL 13-2 Double Diapering with a Stent in Place

A double diapering technique is used to protect the stent (small tube that drains urine) following repair of hypospadias or epispadias.

PROCEDURE

1. Open two diapers on top of each other and place under the infant's perineum.

2. Hold the stent to the side, and place the first diaper over the perineum. Position the stent to drain into the second diaper. Fold the second diaper into place (Figure 13-2).

   RATIONALE: *This process prevents contamination of the stent with feces. Urinary output and urine color can be assessed postsurgery.*

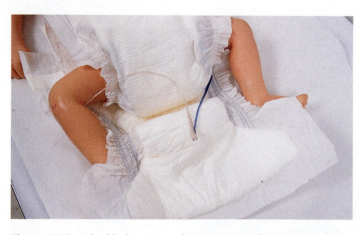

Figure 13-2 *A double diapering technique protects the urinary stent after surgery for hypospadias or epispadias repair. The inner diaper collects stool; the outer diaper, urine.*

Ostomy Care

Ostomies are performed when an infant or child requires fecal or urinary diversion (Figure 13-3). Infants and children may require an ostomy for several reasons, including necrotizing enterocolitis, Hirschsprung disease, imperforate anus, prune-belly syndrome, inflammatory bowel syndrome, spina bifida, tumor, and trauma. An ileostomy, colostomy, or urinary diversion is performed depending on the disorder and its location.

An adhesive appliance is usually applied just after surgery to measure drainage. If a dressing is applied instead of an adhesive appliance, the drainage can be measured by weighing the dressing both before and after saturation. For each 1-g increase in weight of the dressing, approximately 1 mL of fluid has drained into it.

In children and infants, ostomies pose special problems because of the fragility of the skin. Care must be taken to prevent skin breakdown at the site.

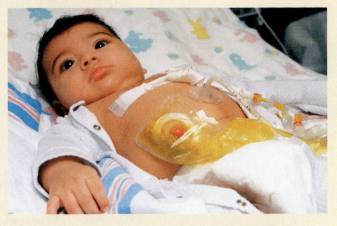

Figure 13-3 *This infant has several gastrointestinal problems and requires ostomies both for gastric feedings and for drainage of fecal material. The care of the skin is challenging and important for this infant so that infection is prevented and adequate nutrition is provided.*

SKILL 13-3 Changing the Dressing for an Infant with an Ostomy

PREPARATION

1. Verify the identity of the child and explain the procedure to the child and parents.

2. Observe drainage on the dressing carefully so it can be described in documentation.

EQUIPMENT AND SUPPLIES

- Gauze
- Tape or other supplies to hold gauze in place

PROCEDURE *Clean Gloves*

1. After each bowel movement, while using gloves, change the dressing, clean and dry the skin, and apply a nonporous substance.
   RATIONALE: *Fecal matter and intestinal fluids, which contain many enzymes, can cause skin breakdown. Measures must be taken to prevent this complication.*

2. Observe the stoma for complications.
   RATIONALE: *Common complications in children include prolapse, retraction, stenosis, and skin breakdown.*

3. To absorb drainage, place gauze with slits cut to fit around the stoma. Use tape to hold the gauze in place. Alternatively, Montgomery straps, an Ace wrap, or a diaper can be used to hold the gauze in place.
   RATIONALE: *Tape sometimes irritates the fragile skin of infants, and other methods could be used to protect the skin.*

NOTE: *Once the stoma has healed and the infant is large enough to wear a pouch, an appliance with a Stomahesive wafer will be used.*

> **CLINICAL TIP**
>
> Avoid adhesive enhancers on the skin of newborns and prematures. Their skin is so thin that removal of the appliance can strip off the skin. Remember that adhesive contains latex, and it should not be used in those who are latex sensitive or allergic.

SKILL 13-4 Changing an Ostomy Pouch for an Infant or Child

PREPARATION

1. Verify the identity of the child and describe or review the procedure with the child and parents.

2. Ask the parents and child about the usual procedures used at home or preferences for changing the ostomy pouch if the child has had the ostomy for some time.

EQUIPMENT AND SUPPLIES

- Pouch and clamp (one piece with adhesive wafer or two pieces with separate pouch and flange and an adhesive wafer)
- Stoma measuring guide
- Stomahesive or other pectin wafer
- Water and washcloth or gauze and cotton balls
- Towel or gauze
- Scissors
- Pads to protect bedding
- Bag for discarding used materials

PROCEDURE *Clean Gloves*

1. Don gloves.

2. Place a pad on the bed to protect it from drainage.

3. Empty the pouch when it is one third to one half full. Remove the pouch, and place it in a sealable plastic bag for disposal.

4. Children will commonly have Stomahesive around the stoma.

   RATIONALE: *This is a wafer of protective material to which a pouch can be attached or from which the pouch can be removed, thus protecting the integrity of the skin. Most wafers need to be changed only once a week.*

5. Wash the skin and the stoma gently with water and soap without oil. Note any skin breakdown or signs of infection. Dry the area.

6. Prepare the new pouch.

7. Measure the Stomahesive or wafer so that it fits exactly around the stoma. Place it securely on the dried skin. Press the pouch firmly against the Stomahesive to form a tight seal. Be careful to avoid making any wrinkles. Close the opening of the pouch with the appropriate clamp.

   RATIONALE: *Measures are taken to prevent fecal matter from leaking onto the skin surface where it could cause breakdown. During the immediate postoperative period the size of the stoma can change, so careful measurement of the wafer to avoid skin damage by fecal material is needed.*

8. Document the procedure, the skin and stoma condition, and how the child tolerated the procedure.

Enemas

There are three important considerations when giving an enema to an infant or a child: the type of fluid, the amount of fluid, and the appropriate distance to insert the tube into the rectum.

Generally, an isotonic fluid such as normal saline is used for children. However, a commercial hypertonic product, such as a pediatric Fleet enema, is sometimes used.

SKILL 13-5 Administering an Enema

PREPARATION

1. Verify the identity of the child and explain the procedure to the child and parents.

2. Assure the child that a bedpan will be kept at the bedside.

3. If the child is toilet trained, place him or her in a bed near a bathroom before giving the enema.

4. Ensure privacy.

EQUIPMENT AND SUPPLIES

- Ordered solution (in container with attached tip) or enema bag and rectal tube (size 14 to 18 French for child; 12 French for infant)
- Water-soluble lubricant
- Pads to protect bedding

PROCEDURE *Clean Gloves*

1. Don gloves.

2. Place absorbent pads on the bed. Position the child on his or her left side, with the knees drawn up to the chest or the right leg flexed over the left leg. You may need an assistant to hold the child in position.
   RATIONALE: *When the child is on the left side, entry of the fluid into the colon is facilitated.*

3. If a rectal tube is being used, attach the solution container, add the fluid, and purge the tubing and tube. Lubricate the tip. If a Fleet enema is being used, the tip is prelubricated.

4. Gently insert the tip to the recommended distance (see Table 13-1). Allow the appropriate volume of fluid to run in slowly, for at least 10 to 15 minutes. If the child complains of cramping, stop the infusion to allow the child to rest, then continue.

5. Infants and children may not be able to retain the fluid. Holding the buttocks together might help.

6. When the child is ready or when it is time to expel the contents of the enema, place the bedpan on the bed or escort the child to the bathroom. Provide privacy as requested. Assess for dizziness or weakness before leaving.

7. Clean the perineum. The child or parent may choose to perform this step.

8. Help the child resume a position of comfort.

9. Assess the enema return for amount and character.

10. Document the procedure, amount and character of enema return, and how the child tolerated the procedure.

TABLE 13-1	Guidelines for Enema Administration to Children	
Age	**Volume (mL)**	**Distance for Inserting Tube**
Infant	40–100	2.5 cm (1 in)
Toddler	100–200	5.0 cm (2 in)
Preschooler	200–300	5.0 cm (2 in)
School-age child	300–500	7.5 cm (3 in)
Adolescent	500–700	10.0 cm (4 in)

14

Skin and Musculoskeletal Care

Skin

SKILL 14-1 Wound Irrigation

Wounds may be irrigated to clean away organisms and dead tissue and to promote healing. Irrigations may be done one time or repeated on a daily or more frequent basis.

PREPARATION

1. Explain the procedure to the child and parent.
2. Perform a pain assessment. See Chapter 10.
   RATIONALE: *The child may need pain medication before the procedure begins to promote comfort.*
3. Place absorbent material under the area.
4. Apply sterile gloves and remove any dressings from the wound.
5. Observe the type and amount of drainage for documentation after the procedure.
6. Discard gloves and wash hands.

EQUIPMENT AND SUPPLIES

- Irrigation solution as ordered. Unless contraindicated the solution should be at room temperature to promote patient comfort.
- Irrigation set or sterile syringes with irrigating tip
- Sterile basin
- Pads for protecting the bedding
- Clean linens
- New topical medications and sterile dressing as ordered

PROCEDURE *Sterile Gloves*

1. Check to be sure that pads and other absorbent materials are adequately positioned under the area to be irrigated.
2. Set up a sterile field and open supplies needed using sterile technique.
3. Apply sterile gloves.
4. Withdraw sterile solution for irrigation.
   RATIONALE: *Solutions are ordered for the ability to clean the area or treat infection. Examples include isotonic saline, Ringer's lactate, and dilute antibiotic solutions.*
5. Release the solution from the syringe, allowing it to flow over the wound. Collect it in a sterile basin under the wound.
6. Repeat several times until the solution is used and/or the wound debris is cleansed.
7. Apply topical medications and dressing as ordered.
8. Clean and dry the child.
9. Clean the field to contain any microorganisms.
10. Document observations of the wound and the child's response to the irrigation.
    RATIONALE: *The condition of the wound and the child's pain level may indicate healing or infection of the wound.*

SKILL 14-2 Burn Wound Care

Children with deep partial-thickness burns often have regular dressing changes and debridement during the healing process. A topical antibiotic cream such as Silvadene is used as a barrier to infectious organisms. Some children have a semipermeable transparent dressing such as Biobrane applied over debrided skin and covered with a gauze dressing. Daily cleansing, debriding, and application of topical antibiotic cream is not performed on burns treated with this type of dressing.

PREPARATION

1. Verify the identity of the child. Explain the procedure and why it is needed to the child and parent. Encourage the parent to provide a distracting activity, such as reading a story or watching a video during the dressing change.

2. Check the physician's orders. Since burn care is a painful procedure, check for pain medication orders and administer medication at least 30 to 60 minutes before starting burn care. Sedation may be used for some debridement procedures.

   RATIONALE: *Medication must be administered so that peak action occurs during the burn dressing change.*

3. Perform hand hygiene. Secure an assistant if needed to position and hold the child and the burned extremity during care.

EQUIPMENT AND SUPPLIES

- Basin
- Sterile normal saline solution
- Large supply of 4 × 4 inch gauze pads
- Forceps
- Scissors
- Sterile tongue blade
- Prescribed topical medication
- Tape
- Absorbent pad

PROCEDURE *Clean and Sterile Gloves*

1. Place the absorbent pad under the area to be cleaned. Put on clean gloves. Soak the wound for about 10 minutes in normal saline solution, or apply a wet dressing to the area. Remove the old dressing. Remove the gloves and perform hand hygiene.

   RATIONALE: *This will soften the wound and make it easier to remove the old dressing.*

2. Using sterile gloves, wash the burn with the gauze pads and sterile normal saline to remove any medication and crusting. Use a firm, circular motion, moving from the inside to the outer edges. Bleeding may occur, but this is a sign of healing, healthy tissue. Rinse with normal saline solution. Pat dry with sterile gauze.

   RATIONALE: *The injured skin secretes serous fluid that forms a tough leathery layer called eschar. This layer must be removed to promote healing.*

3. Some children are placed in a whirlpool bath to soften the eschar and increase circulation.

4. Remove (per physician's orders) any loose or dead skin around the burn's edges by gently lifting it with the forceps and snipping it. This is not painful to the child. Rinse and dry again.

   RATIONALE: *Debridement speeds the healing process.*

5. Place a thin layer of prescribed medication (about 1/8-inch thick) on the burn or gauze with fingers or a sterile tongue blade.

6. Place the medicated gauze on the burn and cover with a dry, sterile dressing.

7. Document the procedure, condition of the burn area, child's pain level, and child's response to the procedure.

SKILL 14-3 Suture and Staple Removal

Skin sutures and staples are used in repairing a wound to hold tissue and skin together. After a period of 1 to 2 weeks, skin healing is adequate and they need to be removed.

Suture Removal

PREPARATION

1. Verify the order.

2. Verify the identity of the child, and explain the procedure to the child and family.

3. Review the patient's history to include date of repair and number of sutures placed.

4. Gather supplies.

EQUIPMENT AND SUPPLIES

- Suture removal kit or sterile forceps and scissors
- Steri-Strips
- Gloves
- Wound cleansing agent according to organization policy

PROCEDURE *Clean Gloves and Sterile Gloves*

1. Perform hand hygiene and apply clean gloves.

2. Remove any dressing covering the sutures. Remove clean gloves, perform hand hygiene, and apply a sterile pair.

3. Assess the wound for healing. If the wound edges are gaping or if there are signs of infection, stop the procedure and consult the physician.
   RATIONALE: *If sutures are removed early, the wound is at risk to reopen. Some approximate adequate preliminary healing times are in Table 14-1.*

TABLE 14-1	Healing Times and Suture Removal Times Common for Various Body Parts
Location of Sutures	**Removal in Days**
Face	5
Chin	5–6
Scalp	7
Trunk	10
Arm/leg	10
Dorsum of hand	10–14
Palm	10–14
Sole	10–14

4. Clean the site with a wound cleansing agent, and gently pat dry with sterile gauze.

5. To remove sutures, using forceps, gently lift the suture knot away from the skin and cut one side of the suture close to the skin.
   RATIONALE: *One cut close to the skin avoids suture material that has been external to be pulled internally as it is removed. It also allows for all the suture material to be removed.*

6. Slowly pull to remove the suture.

7. Remove every other suture. If the wound is healed and not pulling apart, remove the remaining sutures.
   RATIONALE: *Removing every other suture allows for further assessment of wound healing. If the wound is not adequately healed, there should be enough remaining sutures to support the wound during continued healing.*

8. Apply Steri-Strips to the suture line if needed.
   RATIONALE: *Steri-Strips provide additional support as needed.*

9. Remove gloves. Perform hand hygiene. Dispose of gloves and materials in an appropriate manner.

10. Instruct the patient and family regarding further wound care.

11. Document time, number of sutures removed, condition of the wound, and how the patient tolerated the procedure.

Staple Removal

PREPARATION

1. Verify the order.

2. Verify the identity of the child, and explain the procedure to the child and family.

3. Review the patient's history to include date of repair and number of sutures placed.

4. Gather supplies.

EQUIPMENT AND SUPPLIES

- Staple remover
- Steri-Strips
- Clean and sterile gloves
- Wound cleansing agent according to organization policy

PROCEDURE

1. Perform hand hygiene and apply clean gloves.
2. Remove any dressing covering the staples. Remove gloves, perform hand hygiene, and apply a sterile pair.
3. Cleanse the wound according to organization policy.
4. To remove staples: Position a sterile staple remover under the staple to be removed. Squeeze the levers of the staple remover together. The staple will bend in the middle and the edges will pull out.
5. Remove every other staple. If the wound is healed, remove the remaining staples.
   RATIONALE: *Removing every other staple allows for further assessment of wound healing. If the wound is not adequately healed, there should be enough remaining staples to support during continued healing.*
6. Apply Steri-Strips if needed.
   RATIONALE: *Steri-Strips provide additional support as needed.*
7. Remove gloves. Perform hand hygiene. Dispose of gloves and staples/materials in an appropriate manner.
8. Instruct the patient and family regarding further wound care.
9. Document time, number of staples removed, condition of the wound, and how the patient tolerated the procedure.

Casts

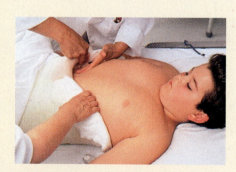

Figure 14-1 *Nurses check the edges of the fresh cast for dryness and rough edges.*

Children often have casts applied after surgery or to treat fractures. They may have white plaster casts that are generally heavy and sturdy. Alternatively, fiberglass casts are lighter and come in various colors, but generally do not last as long. Nurses may assist with cast application and are involved in immediate cast care after application. They commonly instruct the child and family on maintenance of the cast at home. The following procedure describes the nurse's role in care after cast application. See your textbook for further information about management of musculoskeletal treatments (Figure 14-1).

SKILL 14-4 Providing Cast Care

PREPARATION

1. Consult the child's chart for a description of the injury or surgery.

EQUIPMENT AND SUPPLIES

- Cast material (if assisting in application)
- Large basin with water (if assisting in application)
- Pillows with waterproof covering
- Absorbent pads and protectors

PROCEDURE *Clean Gloves*

Following cast application:

1. Elevate a wet cast on pillows covered in plastic.
   RATIONALE: *Elevation decreases edema under the cast which can restrict circulation.*
2. Use the palm of the hands when lifting a wet or damp cast.
   RATIONALE: *Fingertips can indent plaster and create pressure areas.*

NURSING ALERT

Neurovascular impairment under a cast is an emergency. See Skill 6-16. If assessments indicate impaired circulation or neurologic status, notify the physician immediately. Have a cast cutter at the bedside so the cast can quickly be removed if needed and the pressure relieved.

3. Circle and note the date and time of any drainage on the cast.

   RATIONALE: *Some drainage is common after surgery. Monitoring its presence provides clues to the amount and type of fluid lost.*

4. Assess circulation and neurologic status every 15 minutes immediately after surgery or cast placement and then progress to every 30 minutes, 60 minutes, and 2 hours (see Skill 6-16 for further information about neurovascular assessment). Report abnormal findings or changes in condition. Include the following observations on the involved extremities:

   - Distal pulses
   - Capillary refill
   - Color
   - Edema
   - Warmth
   - Movement
   - Sensation
   - Pain, tingling

   RATIONALE: *Circulation and nerves under the cast can be injured if it is too tight.*

5. Use pain-control measures as needed and reassess pain. Report immediately worsening pain or pain that is not controlled by prescribed medication.

6. Check the edges of the cast for roughness or crumbling. Pull the inner stockinette over the edge of the cast and tape once the cast has dried.

   RATIONALE: *These actions can prevent discomfort and skin breakdown.*

7. Keep the cast clean and dry. Cover it with a plastic bag during bathing or toileting.

8. Avoid use of lotions and powders under the cast.

   RATIONALE: *These products can cause skin irritation.*

9. Keep shirts or other clothing over the top edges of casts on young children.

   RATIONALE: *This action helps to prevent the child from placing objects down into the cast which can result in areas of discomfort or skin damage.*

10. Instruct the family about care of the cast at home and when to return for checks and removal of the cast (Table 14-2).

11. Document the cast application, how the child tolerated the procedure, cast care provided, and assessment of vascular and neurologic status.

TABLE 14-2	Instructions for Home Care of the Child with a Cast

Skin Care
- Check the skin around the cast edges for irritation, rubbing, or blistering. The skin should be clean and dry.
- You may cleanse the skin just under the cast edges and between the toes or fingers with a cotton-tipped applicator and rubbing alcohol. Avoid using lotions, oils, and powders near the cast as they may cause caking.
- Avoid poking sharp objects down inside the cast as this may result in injury and infection to the skin.

Cast Care
- Keep the cast dry. Protect plaster with a cast shoe, thick sock, or sling.
- Allow a new, wet cast to air-dry for 24 hours, and maintain good body alignment.
- You may begin walking on a leg cast only if your physician has given you permission to do so.

Be Alert for Possible Complications
- Toes or fingers should be pink, not blue or white.
- Skin should be warm. The tips of the toes should blanch when pinched, with color return within 2 seconds.
- Raise the casted arm or leg above heart level and rest it on pillows to prevent or reduce any swelling.

Notify Your Healthcare Provider If Any of the Following Occur
- Unusual odor beneath the cast
- Tingling
- Burning or numbness in the casted arm or leg
- Drainage through the cast
- Swelling or inability to move the fingers or toes
- Slippage of the cast
- Cast cracked, soft, or loose
- Sudden unexplained fever
- Unusual fussiness or irritability in an infant or child
- Fingers or toes that are blue or white
- Pain that is not relieved by any comfort measures (i.e., repositioning or pain medication)

Courtesy of Shriners Hospital for Children, Spokane, WA. Adapted.

Crutches

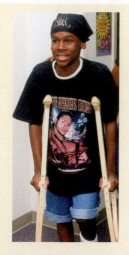

Children may need crutches temporarily after surgery or injury of an extremity, or permanently to assist in ambulation. Crutches are generally supported under the axilla. For long-term use, they may be supported by an attachment fitting over the forearm (Canadian crutches). Nurses assist children to learn to walk safely with crutches, ensure that children using crutches over time are evaluated as needed for correct fit, and monitor the skin that receives pressure from the crutches (Figure 14-2).

Figure 14-2 *This young boy needs to use crutches to walk since he has a non-weight-bearing cast on his left lower leg.*

SKILL 14-5 Setting Crutch Height

PROCEDURE

- While the child is standing, the child's elbows should be slightly and comfortably flexed.
- Place the tip of the crutches about 3 to 6 inches to the upper, outer border of the toes on each foot.
- The upper pad on the crutches should now be lightly placed in the child's axilla.
  RATIONALE: *Crutches that are too high can put pressure on the brachial plexus, causing pain and injury. Crutches that are too low require that the child bend over to walk, and can injure or cause discomfort of the back and neck.*

Braces

Braces are used to treat conditions temporarily (such as for scoliosis in a teenager), or may be used on a long-term basis (such as a child with cerebral palsy who needs leg braces for ambulation). The nurse helps the child accommodate to new braces and then periodically evaluates the fit of the braces and the condition of the skin. Brace wear is usually part of the home and community nursing role. See Table 14-3 for guidelines to teach families about brace wear.

TABLE 14-3   Guidelines for Brace Wear
• Braces should be as comfortable as possible, and the child should have adequate mobility while wearing the brace.
• Begin wearing the brace for periods of 1–2 hours and then progress to 2–4 hours.
• Check the skin at 1- to 2-hour intervals initially, then lengthening to every 4 hours once the skin has been clear for several days. If redness is apparent, leave the brace off and allow the skin to clear. If breakdown has occurred, the brace cannot be worn until healing is complete.
• Always have the child wear a clean white sock, T-shirt, or other thin white liner beneath the brace. Be sure the liner is wrinkle-free under the brace. Avoid using powders or lotions that can cause skin to break down. Toughen any sensitive areas using alcohol wipes on that skin twice daily.
• Reapply the brace when the skin returns to its normal color.
• Return to the physician or orthotic specialist if discomfort or red areas persist or if the brace needs adjustment or repair, or is outgrown.
• Check the brace daily for rough edges.

Traction

A variety of types of traction are used to provide force on bones and muscles. Skin or external traction is sometimes used, whereas skeletal or internal traction involves surgery to place pins into bones which are then attached to traction apparatus. The nurse sets up traction devices as ordered and often applies skin traction with prescribed weights. The nurse also maintains both skin and skeletal traction while providing monitoring of the patient response and condition. See your textbook for further description about types of traction.

SKILL 14-6 Applying and Monitoring Skin Traction

PREPARATION

1. Verify the identity of the child. Explain to the child and family the type of traction and what it will involve.

2. Gather equipment needed and review proper setup.

3. Check the weights to be certain they are the same as those ordered by the physician.

EQUIPMENT AND SUPPLIES

- Poles, pulleys, rope, weight, pads
- Elastic wrap for skin traction

PROCEDURE

1. Set up the prescribed type of traction with proper weights.

2. Apply skin traction as ordered to the particular extremity. Wrap the extremity and apply straps to freely movable prescribed weights.

3. Perform assessments every 30 minutes initially, and then advance to every 1 to 2 hours when stable. Include the following areas:
   - Proper position of traction
   - Proper body alignment
   - Neurovascular status of the extremity (see information on cast care earlier in this chapter and Skill 6-16 on neurovascular assessment)
   - Skin condition under and around the traction application
   - Skin on prominences exposed to the surface of the bed
   - Vital signs
   - Pain and psychologic status

   RATIONALE: *Traction can lead to skin breakdown or neurovascular impairment. Infections can result, especially with internal traction. Regular assessments help to identify problems early. Children may be pulled out of correct alignment by traction and movement in bed and may require frequent repositioning.*

4. Check the child's alignment in bed and reposition as needed.

5. Remove traction according to agency policy, performing assessments and skin care. Reapply as directed in the medical orders.

6. Provide teaching and evaluation of technique if the family will maintain traction at home (Figure 14-3).

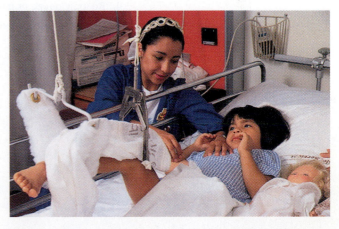

Figure 14-3 *The child in traction needs close monitoring for alignment and proper traction application. Parents can often provide distraction and activities to help the child pass the time during his or her immobility.*

SKILL 14-7 Monitoring Skeletal Traction and Performing Pin Care

PREPARATION

1. Verify orders for the type of traction and amount of weight as well as orders or agency policy regarding pin care.

2. Verify the identity of the child, and explain the procedure to the child and parent.

3. Gather supplies as needed for skin care.

EQUIPMENT AND SUPPLIES

- Sterile gloves (two pairs)
- Sterile applicators
- Normal saline
- Gauze pads

PROCEDURE *Sterile Gloves*

1. Identify that weights are correct and are freely movable. Ropes should be secure and not frayed.

2. Check the child's alignment in bed and reposition as needed.

3. Perform an extremity check as described below and in Skill 6-16, to include the following:

   - Neurovascular status of the extremity (see information on cast care earlier in this chapter)
   - Skin condition under and around the traction application
   - Presence and type of drainage
   - Skin on prominences exposed to the surface of the bed
   - Vital signs
   - Pain and psychologic status

   When pin care is needed, perform the following steps:

1. Perform hand hygiene and don gloves. Remove old gauze from pin sites and assess the condition of the skin and the type of drainage.

2. Remove gloves, perform hand hygiene, open sterile containers so they are readily accessible, and don new gloves.

3. Using sterile technique, cleanse the area around pins with normal saline or other ordered solution. Clean off dried drainage from pins.

   RATIONALE: *Pin care helps to maintain cleanliness and decrease microbial contamination at the insertion sites, and minimizes the chance of infection.*

4. Reapply gauze or pin shields around pin sites.

5. Document assessment findings, the procedure, and the child's responses.

HOME CARE CONSIDERATIONS

Children are increasingly being treated with traction at home. Be certain that the family understands how to set up and maintain the traction. Teach the observations to be made on the extremity involved. Siblings may change the weights or ropes, so close supervision may be needed by parents in some families. A home visit soon after traction begins is often made to evaluate the family's understanding and ability to carry out the regimen.

Appendix A
Physical Growth Charts

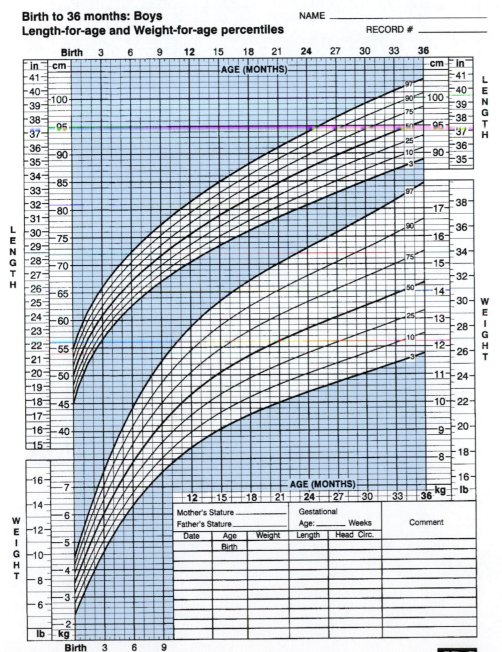

Birth to 36 months: Boys
Length-for-age and Weight-for-age percentiles

NAME _____

RECORD # _____

Figure A-1 *Physical growth percentiles for length and weight—boys: birth to 36 months. From CDC, 2001. www.cdc.gov/growthcharts*

Revised April 20, 2001.
SOURCE: Developed by the National Center for Health Statistics in collaboration with the National Center for Chronic Disease Prevention and Health Promotion (2000).
http://www.cdc.gov/growthcharts

Figure A-2 *Physical growth percentiles for head circumference, weight for length—boys: birth to 36 months.*
From CDC, 2001.
www.cdc.gov/growthcharts

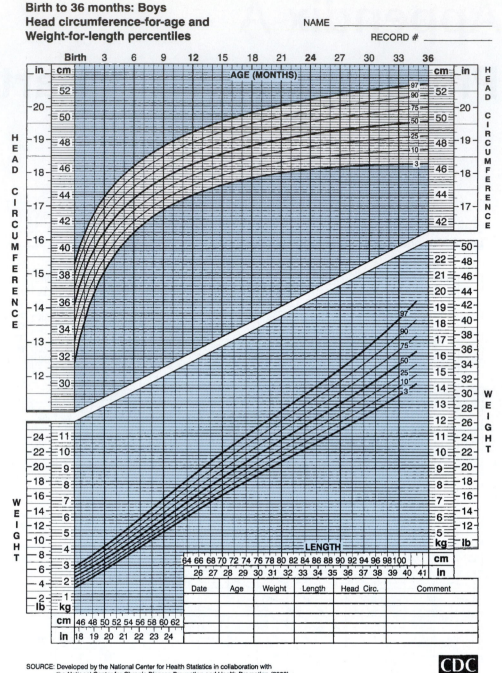

Birth to 36 months: Boys
Head circumference-for-age and
Weight-for-length percentiles

NAME _____

RECORD # _____

SOURCE: Developed by the National Center for Health Statistics in collaboration with
the National Center for Chronic Disease Prevention and Health Promotion (2000).
http://www.cdc.gov/growthcharts

Birth to 36 months: Girls
Length-for-age and Weight-for-age percentiles

NAME _____

RECORD # _____

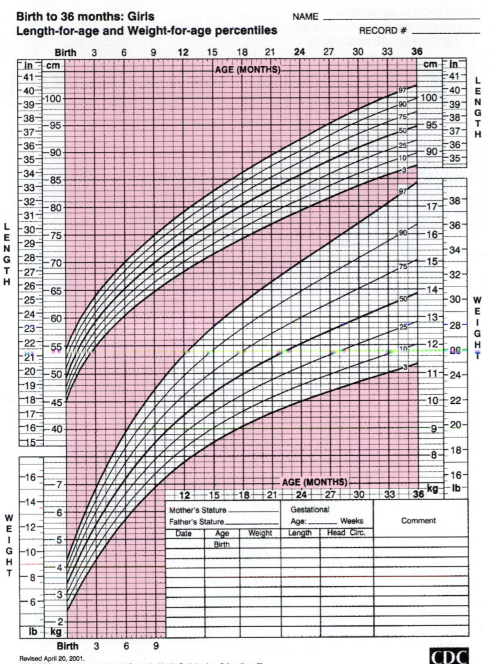

Revised April 20, 2001.

SOURCE: Developed by the National Center for Health Statistics in collaboration with
the National Center for Chronic Disease Prevention and Health Promotion (2000).
http://www.cdc.gov/growthcharts

CDC

Figure A-3 *Physical growth percentiles for length and weight—girls: birth to 36 months.* From CDC, 2001. *www.cdc.gov/growthcharts*

Figure A-4 *Physical growth percentiles for head circumference, weight for length—girls: birth to 36 months.*
From CDC, 2001.
www.cdc.gov/growthcharts

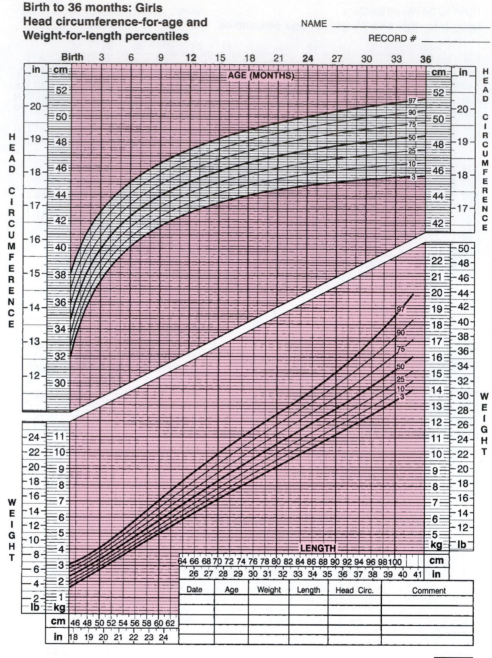

Birth to 36 months: Girls
Head circumference-for-age and
Weight-for-length percentiles

NAME _____

RECORD # _____

SOURCE: Developed by the National Center for Health Statistics in collaboration with
the National Center for Chronic Disease Prevention and Health Promotion (2000).
http://www.cdc.gov/growthcharts

CDC

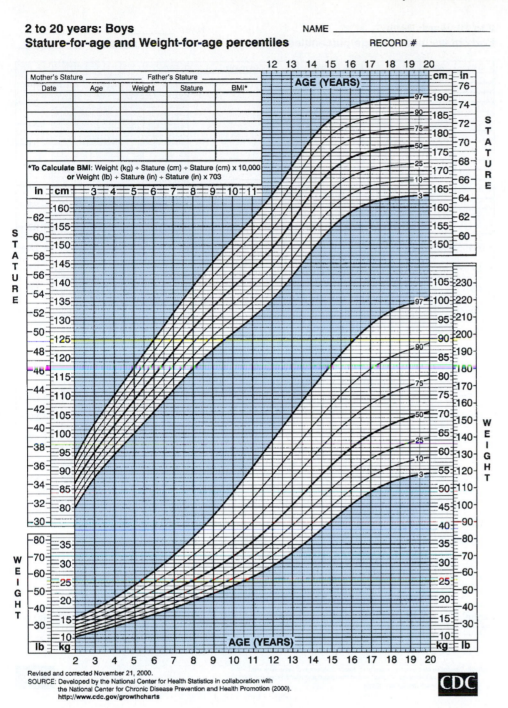

2 to 20 years: Boys
Stature-for-age and Weight-for-age percentiles

NAME _____

RECORD # _____

Figure A-5 *Physical growth percentiles for stature and weight according to age—boys: 2 to 20 years.* From CDC, 2001. *www.cdc.gov/growthcharts*

*To Calculate BMI: Weight (kg) ÷ Stature (cm) ÷ Stature (cm) x 10,000 or Weight (lb) ÷ Stature (in) ÷ Stature (in) x 703

Revised and corrected November 21, 2000.
SOURCE: Developed by the National Center for Health Statistics in collaboration with the National Center for Chronic Disease Prevention and Health Promotion (2000).
http://www.cdc.gov/growthcharts

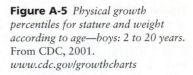

Figure A-6 *Physical growth percentiles for body mass index according to age—boys: 2 to 20 years. From CDC, 2001. www.cdc.gov/growthcharts*

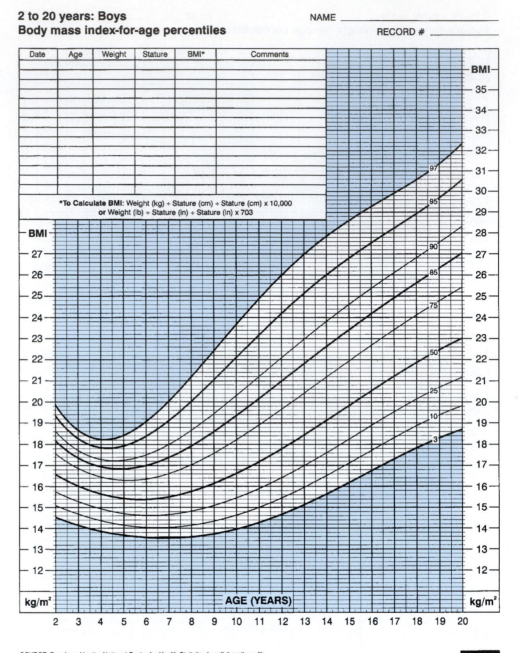

2 to 20 years: Boys
Body mass index-for-age percentiles

NAME _____

RECORD # _____

Date	Age	Weight	Stature	BMI*	Comments

*To Calculate BMI: Weight (kg) ÷ Stature (cm) ÷ Stature (cm) x 10,000
or Weight (lb) ÷ Stature (in) ÷ Stature (in) x 703

AGE (YEARS)

SOURCE: Developed by the National Center for Health Statistics in collaboration with
the National Center for Chronic Disease Prevention and Health Promotion (2000).
http://www.cdc.gov/growthcharts

CDC

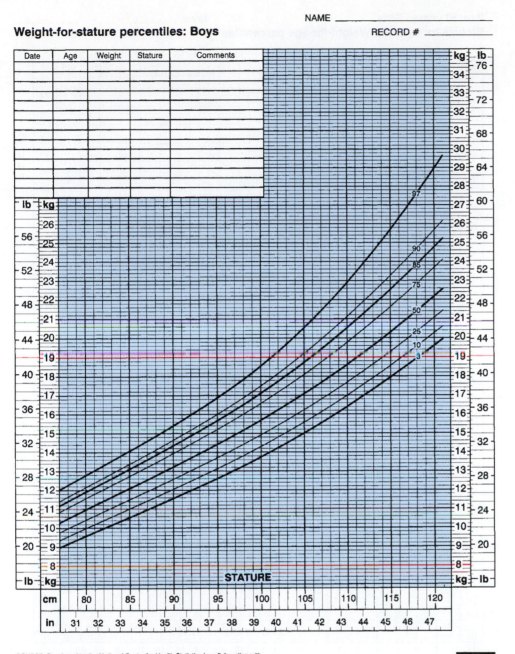

Weight-for-stature percentiles: Boys

NAME _____

RECORD # _____

Date	Age	Weight	Stature	Comments

STATURE

SOURCE: Developed by the National Center for Health Statistics in collaboration with
the National Center for Chronic Disease Prevention and Health Promotion (2000).
http://www.cdc.gov/growthcharts

CDC

Figure A-7 *Physical growth percentiles for weight for stature— boys: 2 to 20 years.*
From CDC, 2001.
www.cdc.gov/growthcharts

Figure A-8 *Physical growth percentiles for stature and weight according to age—girls: 2 to 20 years.* From CDC, 2001. *www.cdc.gov/growthcharts*

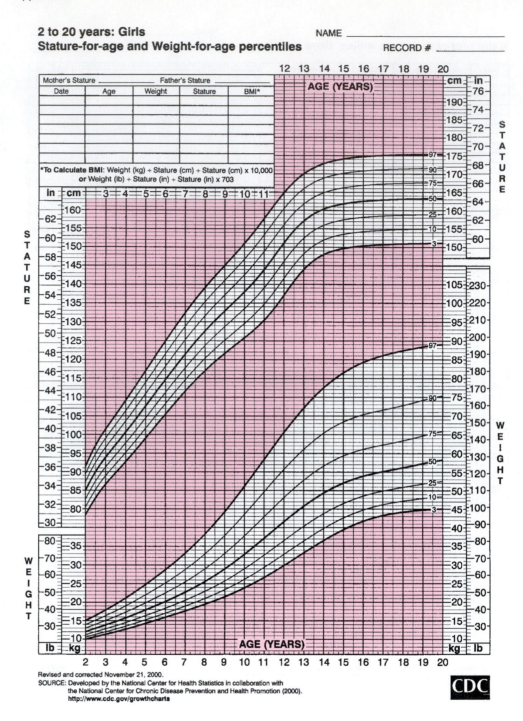

2 to 20 years: Girls
Stature-for-age and Weight-for-age percentiles

NAME _____

RECORD # _____

*To Calculate BMI: Weight (kg) ÷ Stature (cm) ÷ Stature (cm) x 10,000
or Weight (lb) ÷ Stature (in) ÷ Stature (in) x 703

Revised and corrected November 21, 2000.
SOURCE: Developed by the National Center for Health Statistics in collaboration with
the National Center for Chronic Disease Prevention and Health Promotion (2000).
http://www.cdc.gov/growthcharts

CDC

2 to 20 years: Girls
Body mass index-for-age percentiles

NAME _____

RECORD # _____

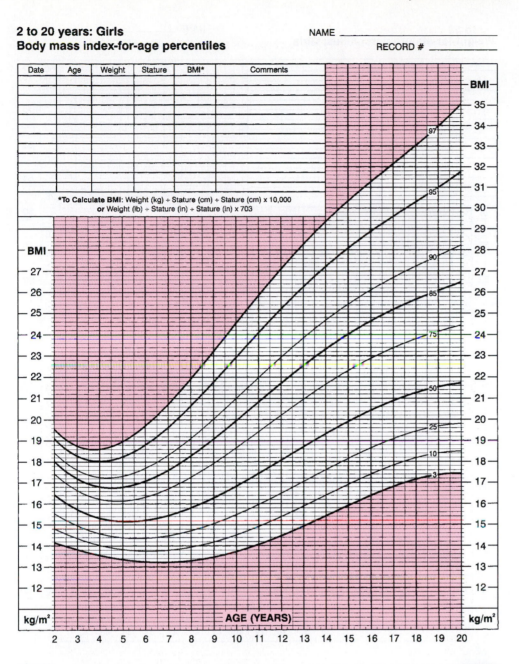

Date	Age	Weight	Stature	BMI*	Comments

*To Calculate BMI: Weight (kg) ÷ Stature (cm) ÷ Stature (cm) x 10,000
or Weight (lb) ÷ Stature (in) ÷ Stature (in) x 703

AGE (YEARS)

SOURCE: Developed by the National Center for Health Statistics in collaboration with
the National Center for Chronic Disease Prevention and Health Promotion (2000).
http://www.cdc.gov/growthcharts

Figure A-9 *Physical growth percentiles for body mass index according to age—girls: 2 to 20 years. From CDC, 2001. www.cdc.gov/growthcharts*

Figure A-10 *Physical growth percentiles for weight for stature—girls: 2 to 20 years.* From CDC, 2001. *www.cdc.gov/growthcharts*

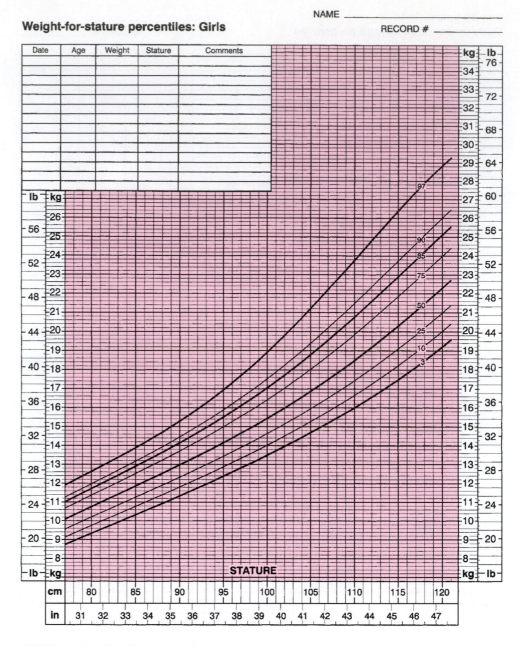

Weight-for-stature percentiles: Girls

NAME _____

RECORD # _____

STATURE

SOURCE: Developed by the National Center for Health Statistics in collaboration with the National Center for Chronic Disease Prevention and Health Promotion (2000). http://www.cdc.gov/growthcharts

CDC

Appendix B

Blood Pressure Values by Age, Sex, and Height Percentiles

BOYS

Blood Pressure Levels for Boys by Age and Height Percentile. Use the child's height percentile for the age and sex from the standard growth charts found in Appendix A. A blood pressure value at 50th percentile for the child's age, sex, and height percentile is considered the midpoint of the normal range. A reading above the 95th percentile indicates hypertension.*

Age (Year)	BP Percentile	Systolic BP (mmHg) Percentile of Height							Diastolic BP (mmHg) Percentile of Height						
		5th	10th	25th	50th	75th	90th	95th	5th	10th	25th	50th	75th	90th	95th
1	50th	00	01	03	05	07	08	09	34	35	36	37	38	39	39
	90th	94	95	97	99	100	102	103	49	50	51	52	53	53	54
	95th	98	99	101	103	104	106	106	54	54	55	56	57	58	58
	99th	105	106	108	110	112	113	114	61	62	63	64	65	66	66
2	50th	84	85	87	88	90	92	92	39	40	41	42	43	44	44
	90th	97	99	100	102	104	105	106	54	55	56	57	58	58	59
	95th	101	102	104	106	108	109	110	59	59	60	61	62	63	63
	99th	109	110	111	113	115	117	117	66	67	68	69	70	71	71
3	50th	86	87	89	91	93	94	95	44	44	45	46	47	48	48
	90th	100	101	103	105	107	108	109	59	59	60	61	62	63	63
	95th	104	105	107	109	110	112	113	63	63	64	65	66	67	67
	99th	111	112	114	116	118	119	120	71	71	72	73	74	75	75
4	50th	88	89	91	93	95	96	97	47	48	49	50	51	51	52
	90th	102	103	105	107	109	110	111	62	63	64	65	66	66	67
	95th	106	107	109	111	112	114	115	66	67	68	69	70	71	71
	99th	113	114	116	118	120	121	122	74	75	76	77	78	78	79
5	50th	90	91	93	95	96	98	98	50	51	52	53	54	55	55
	90th	104	105	106	108	110	111	112	65	66	67	68	69	69	70
	95th	108	109	110	112	114	115	116	69	70	71	72	73	74	74
	99th	115	116	118	120	121	123	123	77	78	79	80	81	81	82
6	50th	91	92	94	96	98	99	100	53	53	54	55	56	57	57
	90th	105	106	108	110	111	113	113	68	68	69	70	71	72	72
	95th	109	110	112	114	115	117	117	72	72	73	74	75	76	76
	99th	116	117	119	121	123	124	125	80	80	81	82	83	84	84
7	50th	92	94	95	97	99	100	101	55	55	56	57	58	59	59
	90th	106	107	109	111	113	114	115	70	70	71	72	73	74	74
	95th	110	111	113	115	117	118	119	74	74	75	76	77	78	78
	99th	117	118	120	122	124	125	126	82	82	83	84	85	86	86
8	50th	94	95	97	99	100	102	102	56	57	58	59	60	60	61
	90th	107	109	110	112	114	115	116	71	72	72	73	74	75	76
	95th	111	112	114	116	118	119	120	75	76	77	78	79	79	80
	99th	119	120	122	123	125	127	127	83	84	85	86	87	87	88
9	50th	95	96	98	100	102	103	104	57	58	59	60	61	61	62
	90th	109	110	112	114	115	117	118	72	73	74	75	76	76	77
	95th	113	114	116	118	119	121	121	76	77	78	79	80	81	81
	99th	120	121	123	125	127	128	129	84	85	86	87	88	88	89

BOYS

Blood Pressure Levels for Boys by Age and Height Percentile. Use the child's height percentile for the age and sex from the standard growth charts found in Appendix A. A blood pressure value at 50th percentile for the child's age, sex, and height percentile is considered the midpoint of the normal range. A reading above the 95th percentile indicates hypertension.*—*Continued*

Age (Year)	BP Percentile	Systolic BP (mmHg) Percentile of Height							Diastolic BP (mmHg) Percentile of Height						
		5th	10th	25th	50th	75th	90th	95th	5th	10th	25th	50th	75th	90th	95th
10	50th	97	98	100	102	103	105	106	58	59	60	61	61	62	63
	90th	111	112	114	115	117	119	119	73	73	74	75	76	77	78
	95th	115	116	117	119	121	122	123	77	78	79	80	81	81	82
	99th	122	123	125	127	128	130	130	85	86	86	88	88	89	90
11	50th	99	100	102	104	105	107	107	59	59	60	61	62	63	63
	90th	113	114	115	117	119	120	121	74	74	75	76	77	78	78
	95th	117	118	119	121	123	124	125	78	78	79	80	81	82	82
	99th	124	125	127	129	130	132	132	86	86	87	88	89	90	90
12	50th	101	102	104	106	108	109	110	59	60	61	62	63	63	64
	90th	115	116	118	120	121	123	123	74	75	75	76	77	78	79
	95th	119	120	122	123	125	127	127	78	79	80	81	82	82	83
	99th	126	127	129	131	133	134	135	86	87	88	89	90	90	91
13	50th	104	105	106	108	110	111	112	60	60	61	62	63	64	64
	90th	117	118	120	122	124	125	126	75	75	76	77	78	79	79
	95th	121	122	124	126	128	129	130	79	79	80	81	82	83	83
	99th	128	130	131	133	135	136	137	87	87	88	89	90	91	91
14	50th	106	107	109	111	113	114	115	60	61	62	63	64	65	65
	90th	120	121	123	125	126	128	128	75	76	77	78	79	79	80
	95th	124	125	127	128	130	132	132	80	80	81	82	83	84	84
	99th	131	132	134	136	138	139	140	87	88	89	90	91	92	92
15	50th	109	110	112	113	115	117	117	61	62	63	64	65	66	66
	90th	122	124	125	127	129	130	131	76	77	78	79	80	80	81
	95th	126	127	129	131	133	134	135	81	81	82	83	84	85	85
	99th	134	135	136	138	140	142	142	88	89	90	91	92	93	93
16	50th	111	112	114	116	118	119	120	63	63	64	65	66	67	67
	90th	125	126	128	130	131	133	134	78	78	79	80	81	82	82
	95th	129	130	132	134	135	137	137	82	83	83	84	85	86	87
	99th	136	137	139	141	143	144	145	90	90	91	92	93	94	94
17	50th	114	115	116	118	120	121	122	65	66	66	67	68	69	70
	90th	127	128	130	132	134	135	136	80	80	81	82	83	84	84
	95th	131	132	134	136	138	139	140	84	85	86	87	87	88	89
	99th	139	140	141	143	145	146	147	92	93	93	94	95	96	97

BP, blood pressure

*The 90th percentile is 1.28 SD, 95th percentile is 1.645 SD, and the 99th percentile is 2.326 SD over the mean.

National Heart, Lung, and Blood Institute. (2004). Blood pressure tables for children and adolescents from the fourth report on the diagnosis, evaluation, and treatment of high blood pressure in children and adolescents. *www.nhlbi.nih.gov/guidelines/hypertension/child_tbl.htm,* accessed 6/11/2004.

GIRLS

Blood Pressure Levels for Girls by Age and Height Percentile. Use the child's height percentile for the age and sex from the standard growth charts found in Appendix A. A blood pressure value at 50th percentile for the child's age, sex, and height percentile is considered the midpoint of the normal range. A reading above the 95th percentile indicates hypertension.*

Age (Year)	BP Percentile	Systolic BP (mmHg) Percentile of Height							Diastolic BP (mmHg) Percentile of Height						
		5th	10th	25th	50th	75th	90th	95th	5th	10th	25th	50th	75th	90th	95th
1	50th	83	84	85	86	88	89	90	38	39	39	40	41	41	42
	90th	97	97	98	100	101	102	103	52	53	53	54	55	55	56
	95th	100	101	102	104	105	106	107	56	57	57	58	59	59	60
	99th	108	108	109	111	112	113	114	64	64	65	65	66	67	67
2	50th	85	85	87	88	89	91	91	43	44	44	45	46	46	47
	90th	98	99	100	101	103	104	105	57	58	58	59	60	61	61
	95th	102	103	104	105	107	108	109	61	62	62	63	64	65	65
	99th	109	110	111	112	114	115	117	69	69	70	70	71	72	72
3	50th	86	87	88	89	91	92	93	47	48	48	49	50	50	51
	90th	100	100	102	103	104	106	106	61	62	62	63	64	64	65
	95th	104	104	105	107	108	109	110	65	66	66	67	68	68	69
	99th	111	111	113	114	115	116	117	73	73	74	74	75	76	76
4	50th	88	88	90	91	92	94	94	50	50	51	52	52	53	54
	90th	101	102	103	104	106	107	108	64	64	65	66	67	67	68
	95th	105	106	107	108	110	111	112	68	68	69	70	71	71	72
	99th	112	113	114	115	117	118	119	76	76	76	77	78	79	79
5	50th	89	90	91	93	94	95	96	52	53	53	54	55	55	56
	90th	103	103	105	106	107	109	109	66	67	67	68	69	69	70
	95th	107	107	108	110	111	112	113	70	71	71	72	73	73	74
	99th	114	114	116	117	118	120	120	78	78	79	79	80	81	81
6	50th	91	92	93	94	96	97	98	54	54	55	56	56	57	58
	90th	104	105	106	108	109	110	111	68	68	69	70	70	71	72
	95th	108	109	110	111	113	114	115	72	72	73	74	74	75	76
	99th	115	116	117	119	120	121	122	80	80	80	81	82	83	83
7	50th	93	93	95	96	97	99	99	55	56	56	57	58	58	59
	90th	106	107	108	109	111	112	113	69	70	70	71	72	72	73
	95th	110	111	112	113	115	116	116	73	74	74	75	76	76	77
	99th	117	118	119	120	122	123	124	81	81	82	82	83	84	84
8	50th	95	95	96	98	99	100	101	57	57	57	58	59	60	60
	90th	108	109	110	111	113	114	114	71	71	71	72	73	74	74
	95th	112	112	114	115	116	118	118	75	75	75	76	77	78	78
	99th	119	120	121	122	123	125	125	82	82	83	83	84	85	86
9	50th	96	97	98	100	101	102	103	58	58	58	59	60	61	61
	90th	110	110	112	113	114	116	116	72	72	72	73	74	75	75
	95th	114	114	115	117	118	119	120	76	76	76	77	78	79	79
	99th	121	121	123	124	125	127	127	83	83	84	84	85	86	87

(continued)

GIRLS

Blood Pressure Levels for Girls by Age and Height Percentile. Use the child's height percentile for the age and sex from the standard growth charts found in Appendix A. A blood pressure value at 50th percentile for the child's age, sex, and height percentile is considered the midpoint of the normal range. A reading above the 95th percentile indicates hypertension.*—*Continued*

Age (Year)	BP Percentile	Systolic BP (mmHg) Percentile of Height							Diastolic BP (mmHg) Percentile of Height						
		5th	10th	25th	50th	75th	90th	95th	5th	10th	25th	50th	75th	90th	95th
10	50th	98	99	100	102	103	104	105	59	59	59	60	61	62	62
	90th	112	112	114	115	116	118	118	73	73	73	74	75	76	76
	95th	116	116	117	119	120	121	122	77	77	77	78	79	80	80
	99th	123	123	125	126	127	129	129	84	84	85	86	86	87	88
11	50th	100	101	102	103	105	106	107	60	60	60	61	62	63	63
	90th	114	114	116	117	118	119	120	74	74	74	75	76	77	77
	95th	118	118	119	121	122	123	124	78	78	78	79	80	81	81
	99th	125	125	126	128	129	130	131	85	85	86	87	87	88	89
12	50th	102	103	104	105	107	108	109	61	61	61	62	63	64	64
	90th	116	116	117	119	120	121	122	75	75	75	76	77	78	78
	95th	119	120	121	123	124	125	126	79	79	79	80	81	82	82
	99th	127	127	128	130	131	132	133	86	86	87	88	88	89	90
13	50th	104	105	106	107	109	110	110	62	62	62	63	64	65	65
	90th	117	118	119	121	122	123	124	76	76	76	77	78	79	79
	95th	121	122	123	124	126	127	128	80	80	80	81	82	83	83
	99th	128	129	130	132	133	134	135	87	87	88	89	89	90	91
14	50th	106	106	107	109	110	111	112	63	63	63	64	65	66	66
	90th	119	120	121	122	124	125	125	77	77	77	78	79	80	80
	95th	123	123	125	126	127	129	129	81	81	81	82	83	84	84
	99th	130	131	132	133	135	136	136	88	88	89	90	90	91	92
15	50th	107	108	109	110	111	113	113	64	64	64	65	66	67	67
	90th	120	121	122	123	125	126	127	78	78	78	79	80	81	81
	95th	124	125	126	127	129	130	131	82	82	82	83	84	85	85
	99th	131	132	133	134	136	137	138	89	89	90	91	91	92	93
16	50th	108	108	110	111	112	114	114	64	64	65	66	66	67	68
	90th	121	122	123	124	126	127	128	78	78	79	80	81	81	82
	95th	125	126	127	128	130	131	132	82	82	83	84	85	85	86
	99th	132	133	134	135	137	138	139	90	90	90	91	92	93	93
17	50th	108	109	110	111	113	114	115	64	65	65	66	67	67	68
	90th	122	122	123	125	126	127	128	78	79	79	80	81	81	82
	95th	125	126	127	129	130	131	132	82	83	83	84	85	85	86
	99th	133	133	134	136	137	138	139	90	90	91	91	92	93	93

BP, blood pressure

*The 90th percentile is 1.28 SD, 95th percentile is 1.645 SD, and the 99th percentile is 2.326 SD over the mean.

National Heart, Lung, and Blood Institute. (2004). Blood pressure tables for children and adolescents from the fourth report on the diagnosis, evaluation, and treatment of high blood pressure in children and adolescents. *www.nhlbi.nih.gov/guidelines/hypertension/child_tbl.htm*, accessed 6/11/2004.

Appendix C
West Nomogram—Body Surface Area

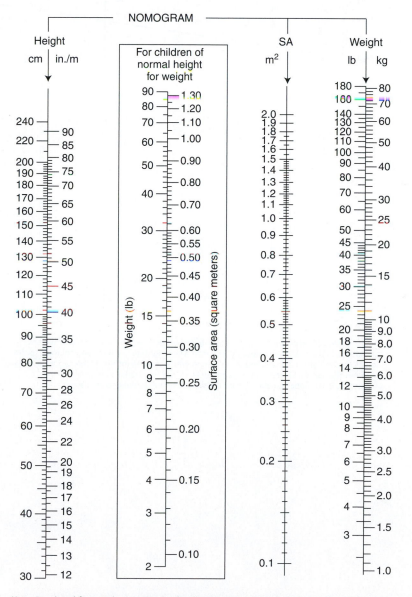

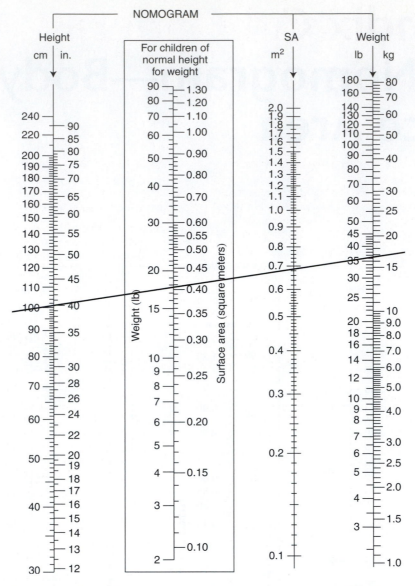

Pediatric doses of medications are generally based on body surface area (BSA) or weight. To calculate a child's BSA, draw a straight line from the height (in the left-hand column) to the weight (in the right-hand column). The point at which the line intersects the surface area (SA) column is the BSA (measured in square meters [m^2]). If the child is of roughly normal proportion, BSA can be calculated from the weight alone (in the enclosed area).

Citations and General References

Adirim, T. A., Smith, E., & Singh, T. (2006). *SCOPE: Special children's outreach and prehospital education.* Sudbury, MA: Jones & Bartlett.

American Heart Association Emergency Cardiovascular Care Committee. (2005). American Heart Association 2005 Guidelines for cardiopulmonary resuscitation and emergency cardiovascular care. *Circulation,* 112 [Suppl I, IV-1 to IV-5].

Bell, E. F. (n.d.). *Iowa neonatology handbook: Pulmonary sampling techniques for arterial blood gas samples.* Retrieved October 7, 2005, from *http://vh.org/pediatric/provider/pediatrics/iowa neonatologyhandbook/pulmonary/samplingbloodgas.html.*

Bindler, R. M., & Howry, L. B. (2005). *Pediatric drug guide and nursing implications.* Upper Saddle River, NJ: Prentice Hall Health.

Borkowski, S. (2005, May). Irritation, redness, and drainage at the site of a pediatric gastrostomy. *Clinical Advisor,* 90–91.

Boyce, J. M., & Pittet, D. (2002). Guideline for hand hygiene in health-care settings: Recommendations of the Healthcare Infection Control Practices Advisory Committee and the HICPAC/SHEA/APIC/IDSA hand hygiene task force. *Infection Control and Hospital Epidemiology, 23,* S3–S40.

Burd, A., & Burd, R. S. (2003). The who, what, why and how-to guide for gastrostomy tube placement in infants. *Advances in Neonatal Care, 3,* 197–205.

Craig, J. V., Lancaster, G. A., Taylor, S., Williamson, P. R., & Smyth, R. L. (2002). Infrared ear thermometry compared with rectal thermometry in children: A systemic review. *Lancet, 360*(9333), 603–609.

Dieckmann, R., & American Academy of Pediatrics. (2006). *Pediatric education for prehospital professionals.* (2nd ed.). Sudbury, MA: Jones & Bartlett.

Falzon, A., Grech, V., Caruana, B., et al. (2003). How reliable is axillary temperature measurement? *Acta Paediatrica, 92,* 309–313.

Fiske, E. (2004). Effective strategies to prepare infants and families for home tracheostomy care. *Advances in Neonatal Care, 4*(1), 42–53.

Galley, R. (2005). Understanding pulse oximetry. *Clinician Reviews, 15*(10), 32–36.

Goodfellow, L. T., & Jones, M. (2002). Bronchial hygiene therapy: From traditional hands-on techniques to modern technological approaches. *American Journal of Nursing, 102*(1), 37–43.

Gracey, K., Burd, A., & Burd, R. (2003). Guide for home gastrostomy tube care. *Advances in Neonatal Care, 3,* 206–207.

Guido, G. W. (2006). *Legal & ethical issues in nursing* (4th ed.). Upper Saddle River, NJ: Prentice Hall Health.

Holmes, S. (2004). Enteral feeding and percutaneous endoscopic gastrostomy. *Nursing Standard, 18*(20), 41–43.

Huffman, S., Jarczyk, K. S., O'Brien, E., Pieper, P., & Bayne, A. (2004). Methods to confirm feeding tube placement: Application of research in practice. *Pediatric Nursing, 30,* 10–13.

Johnson, L. (1999). Factors known to raise intracranial pressure and the associated implications for nursing management. *Nursing in Critical Care, 3,* 117–120.

Kee, J. L. (2005). *Laboratory and diagnostic tests with nursing implications* (7th ed.). Upper Saddle River, NJ: Pearson Prentice Hall.

Ladewig, P. W., London, M. L., & Davidson, M. R. (2006). *Contemporary maternal-newborn care* (6th ed.). Upper Saddle River, NJ: Prentice Hall.

Lewarski, J. S. (2005). Long-term care of the patient with a tracheostomy. *Respiratory Care, 50*(4), 534–537.

Maccioli, G. A., Dorman, T., Brown, B. R., Mazuski, J. E., McLean, B. A., Kuszaj, J. M., et al. (2003). Clinical practice guidelines for the maintenance of patient physical safety in the intensive care unit: Use of restraining therapies—American College of Critical Care Medicine Task Force 2001–2002. *Critical Care Medicine, 31,* 2665–2676.

Mitchell, A., & Waltman, P. A. (2003). Oral sucrose and pain relief in preterm infants. *Pain Management Nursing, 4*(2), 62–69.

National Center for Infectious Diseases. (2002). Guidelines for the prevention of intravascular catheter-related infections. *Morbidity and Mortality Weekly Report, 51*(RR10), 1–26.

Popovich, D. M., Richiuso, N., & Danek, G. (2004). Pediatric health care providers' knowledge of pulse oximetry. *Pediatric Nursing, 30*(1), 14–20.

Radeos, M. S., & Camargo, C. A. (2004). Predicted peak expiratory flow: Differences across formulae in the literature. *American Journal of Emergency Medicine, 22*(7), 516–521.

Robertson, J., & Shilkofski, N. (2005). *Harriet Lane handbook.* (17th ed.). Philadelphia: Elsevier Mosby.

Stebor, A. D. (2005). Basic principles of noninvasive blood pressure measurement in infants. *Advances in Neonatal Care, 5*(5), 252–261.

Tillett, J. (2005). Adolescents and informed consent: Ethical and legal issues. *Journal of Perinatal and Neonatal Nursing, 19,* 112–121.

Wong, D. L., & Baker, C. M. (1988). Pain in children: Comparison of assessment scales. *Pediatric Nursing, 14,* 9-16.

Index